ST BARNABAS HOSPICE
WORTHING
— A History —

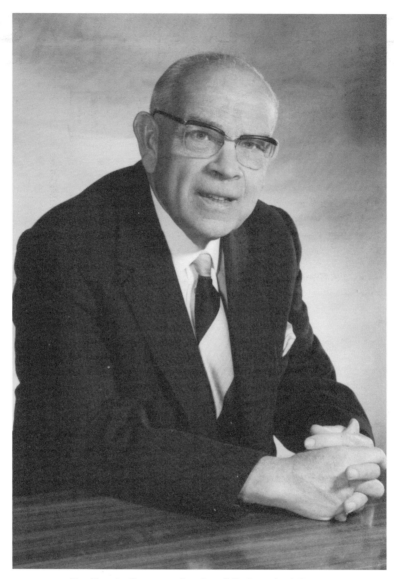

Dr. Francis Gusterson, founder of St Barnabas' Hospice

ST BARNABAS' HOSPICE
WORTHING

— A History —

David S. Farrant

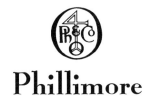

Phillimore

1998

Published by
PHILLIMORE & CO. LTD.
Shopwyke Manor Barn, Chichester, West Sussex

© D.S. Farrant, 1998

ISBN 0 85033 971 5

Printed and bound in Great Britain by
REDWOOD BOOKS
Trowbridge, Wiltshire

To Gus

CONTENTS

List of Illustrations viii
Preface ix
Foreword: Lady Sarah Clutton xi

1   The Promised Land 1
2   The Caring Begins 13
3   The Mission 24
4   Expansion 35
5   Centre of Excellence 45

Appendix I 55
Appendix II 56
Appendix III 58

Index 59

LIST OF ILLUSTRATIONS

Frontispiece: Dr. Francis Gusterson

1. Squadron Leader Gusterson with the R.A.F. in India.................. 2
2. Newspaper appeal... 7
3. The Mayor of Worthing initiates the construction work.............. 9
4. Mr. Harry Bunce and Dr. Gusterson, 1972 11
5. The gift of two King's Fund beds from Worthing Companions Club... 14
6. Presentation of cheque from West Nova Scotia Regiment 16
7. The Duchess of Roxburghe opens the St Barnabas' Nursing Home.... 20
8. Presentation by Miss Stroud to Miss Sackse on her retirement 27
9. Lavinia, Duchess of Norfolk during a visit 28
10. Letter of condolence from the Duchess of Norfolk 34
11. Dr. Kingsbury by the fish-pond 37
12. Derek Jameson presents a cheque 41
13. Diana, Princess of Wales, meets a group of volunteers.............. 44
14. The first shop, Rowlands Road, Worthing 47
15. Dr. Adrian Ruddle, appointed Medical Director, 1993.............. 48
16. Lavinia, the President, makes friends with 'Brigadier' the shire horse .. 49
17. 'Aldaniti' – star guest at the fête 50
18. The 'Batman' float, Worthing Carnival, 1994 51
19. Cosworth, the cat.. 53
20. Martyn Lewis gives the address at the 25th Anniversary Service 54

Front cover: Icon of St Barnabas painted by local Christian artist Gary Bevans, given by the family of Jacky Novak.

PREFACE

In the 1970s, when I was Honorary Secretary of the Readers' Board in the Diocese of Chichester, I came to know Dr. Gusterson, then Lay Reader at Thakeham. At a time when the concept of hospices was in its infancy, he used to talk about his vision of building a home in Worthing for patients with a terminal illness.

Our paths separated, but when I came to Worthing I soon discovered, through my pastoral visiting, that Gus' vision had become a reality. When Alan Welton, the General Manager of St Barnabas' asked me if I would like to write a history of the first 25 years, I was keen to respond, and it has been a real pleasure to see how Dr. Gusterson realised that vision.

Many people have helped me along the way to produce this little book. 38 members of the Association of St Barnabas' took time to write to me about their reminiscences; these have been fundamental in understanding the ethos of the Hospice. My endless questions to past officers and others were handled patiently and kindly, among them Mrs. Jill Annis, Mrs. Patricia Bowles, Mr. John Brenton, Mr. Wilfred East, the Revd Hugh Ford, Mr. Ken Hammond, Mrs. Joan Hunter, Mr. Peter Lock, and Mr. Burnham Roe.

I am most grateful to Dr. Gusterson's daughter, Mrs. Jane Harvey-Samuel and her husband, John, for information about his early career and for loaning photographs. Also to Mr. Edward Kellett of Guild Care who was a most helpful source of information about the formative years. The staff of the *Worthing Herald* very kindly supplied press-cuttings and photographs and gave permission for their publication.

I wish to thank Dr. Alan Kingsbury, Dr. Adrian Ruddle and Miss Margaret Stroud who read the typescript and suggested corrections and alterations and without whose advice this history would have been seriously weakened.

To the staff of St Barnabas' I express my thanks for their response to my requests for documents and information, especially Mrs. Penny Eggebrecht, Mrs. Anne Ewens, Mrs. Wendy Gaylor, Mrs. Stella Mason, Mrs. Pat Read, and Mrs. Joy Watts. My thanks, too, to Mrs. Pauline Heatherington who, as fund-raiser, was a constant support; Alan Welton was a source of sound advice and proved he knows how to oil all the necessary wheels. My thanks to Noel Osborne, Managing Director of Phillimore & Co. Ltd. who has been so supportive of this first book on a hospice which he has published. In the writing and preparation, Nicola Willmot has, once again, accepted with equanimity the ideas and questions which an amateur always presents to a professional, not least in the publishing field.

Any errors or omissions in this book are entirely mine. If it gives glory to its founder, expresses gratitude to those who have worked to achieve his vision and encourages those who are responsible for its future, then it will have achieved its aim.

DAVID FARRANT

Philosophy

St Barnabas' Hospice is more than just a building.

It is a service that seeks to provide continuing care to encourage and enable people to live to the limits of their horizons, even when their illness cannot be cured.

Each one of us, as patient, staff, family, volunteer or friend is a unique individual within a caring team. We are committed to work to the best of our ability to relieve that distress which comes with the realisation of our mortality.

We are mutually dependent on one another, sharing in our difficulties and distress and seeking to be supported by each other's strengths and skills.

THE DOVER
POLING, ARUNDEL
WEST SUSSEX BN18 9PX

Over 30 years ago, it was proposed to build a Home for cancer patients in Worthing. The man who accepted that challenging task, Dr. Francis Gusterson, was a local GP and then anaesthetist at Worthing Hospital. He was a man with a vision. His strong Christian faith shone out in his dedication to those in his care. His determination to succeed, his humility in achievement and his missionary zeal are the hallmarks of his work for St Barnabas' Hospice, which opened its doors on 1 January 1973.

My father, Bernard, was the first President and he was succeeded by my mother, Lavinia. I feel very honoured to have been asked to be the next President carrying on the family link. We all greatly admired 'Gus' as he was affectionately known. St Barnabas' has grown in both scope and size and yet retains its unique family atmosphere, especially in the loving care shown by the medical and nursing staff.

The record of past achievements in providing comfort, care and consolation shows that St Barnabas' has a vision for the future, as well as being a fitting memorial to its founder in this its 25th anniversary year.

Lady Sarah Clutton
President

CHAPTER 1

THE PROMISED LAND

'Any attempt to define the precise beginning of St Barnabas' Home is rather like searching for the source of a river. There is rarely one actual source – usually a large collecting area is involved. Many small streams of equal significance are the real source'.

That is how Dr. Gusterson, the Founder of St Barnabas', began his booklet about the first five years of its history. Nevertheless, there are some well documented sources which show how the need was identified.

Within the Worthing Group Hospital area in 1965, there were 714 deaths from cancer, of which about 440 occurred either at home or in commercial nursing homes. Around 70 per cent of the deaths were in the Worthing borough and rural district. The man who spotted the importance of these figures was Dr. R.B. Franks, consultant geriatrician to the group. Dr. Franks had first become aware of the need in 1962 when there had been 651 deaths in the area. The yearly increase of 10 per cent was, to him, an alarming factor as far as the care of the terminally ill was concerned. Unless some major breakthrough happened in the prevention and treatment of cancer, the need would become overwhelming.

His proposed solution was to establish a terminal home for cancer patients which would cater for their spiritual as well as their physical needs. He felt that public support for such a home would be 'on a generous scale' though support from statutory sources would be required, especially regarding maintenance costs in the early years.

At the same time, the trustees of the Worthing Remembrance Fund were concerned about the use and volume of the gifts they were receiving. The fund, originally called the Flower Fund, had been set up under the umbrella of the Council for Social Service (now known as Guild Care). The Fund was 'for those people or their relatives who decide that at funerals they prefer not to have floral tributes but to invite those who wish to pay homage to send a donation to the Remembrance Fund so that it may be given to good causes'. The trustees were finding it difficult to allocate the monies received in any meaningful way. They felt that the funds would be much healthier if a specific project or need could be addressed; donors were naturally wary about giving to unspecific aims.

In November 1966 Mr. Joseph Sayers, Clerk to the trustees of the Fund, telephoned the honorary medical officer of the Caer Gwent Nursing Home, Dr. F.R. Gusterson to say that the trustees of the Remembrance Fund had decided, after discussions with Dr. Franks, that the money given to them would be better used if it were allocated to a specific project. Dr. Franks had mentioned the need for a home for patients in the terminal stages of cancer; would Dr. Gusterson take on the chairmanship of such an appeal to build a home in Worthing?

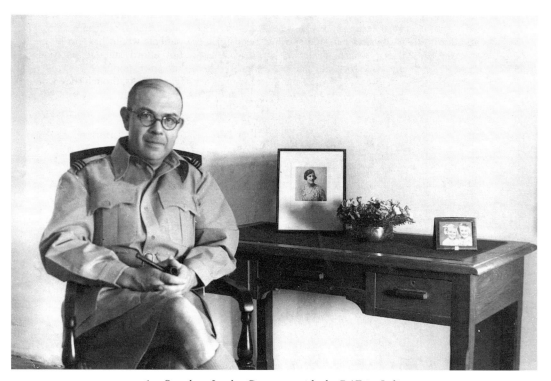

1 *Squadron Leader Gusterson with the RAF in India*

His response is interesting: 'Needless to say, I demurred, knowing what an enormous task this would be'.

So who was this doctor whom the trustees thought would be the ideal person for this project?

Francis Roy Gusterson was born in Tunbridge Wells on 15 January 1906. He was brought up in London, his father being a Baptist Minister in Streatham. He received his medical training at St Thomas' Hospital, qualifying as MRCS, LRCP and graduating three years later MB and BS. He entered general practice in Worthing, his surgery overlooking Broadwater Green. During the war he served in the RAF as a Squadron Leader and was drafted to Karachi and then Bombay. After the war he returned to Worthing and became a full-time consultant anaesthetist. 'Gus', as he was affectionately known to all his friends and colleagues, took a lively interest in charity work. He became a member of the Round Table in 1931 and the Rotary Club in 1946. He was a member of the Executive of Worthing Council of Social Service and for many years chairman of 'The Priory', one of the Field Lane Institute Homes for the Elderly in Worthing. He also was a keen member of the committee of Worthing Boys' Club, taking a special interest in their boxing. He married Dorothy Frampton, who was to give him so much quiet, strong support in his very active life.

This was the man in whom the idea lodged and would not go away. Early in 1967 he met the Borough Treasurer, Mr. Herbert Keeling and Mr. Sayers with another of the trustees. Then, he says, 'a possible scheme began to emerge'. It was:

To build a purpose-built home for about 30 patients in the terminal stages of illness.

In addition to their physical care the spiritual needs of these patients would have to be met.

That the first concern would be for patients who could not afford suitable alternative accommodation, though any suitable patient would be eligible for admission.

That this Home would be entirely independent of any other organisations, though they would be asked to help.

These terms were agreed by the trustees and Dr. Gusterson was asked to form a special committee. He wrote: 'I had no option but to accept the challenge'.

He felt that he needed people who, because of their experience, could offer sound advice as well as ideas. It was important that they should not be already too involved in other affairs in the town and that they would unreservedly accept the main principles laid down. He wanted them to think very carefully before accepting any invitation to join the committee. These were its members:

Treasurer: Burnham W.F. Roe, Manager, National Provincial Bank, Worthing.
Legal Adviser: Richard V. Stapleton, solicitor.
Dr. Raymond Franks, Consultant in Geriatrics to the Worthing Group Hospitals.
Canon Joseph W. Reeves, Vicar of Ferring and Rural Dean of Worthing.
Revd Hubert Janisch, Minister of Christchurch Road Baptist Church and at that time Moderator of the National Federal Free Church Council
Alderman Mrs. Harriet M. Peryer.
Councillor Mrs. Nancy Lephard, at that time Chairman of the Health Committee.
Herbert Keeling, Borough Treasurer of Worthing.
James Bedford, chartered surveyor.
Ernest Manley Bird, company director and Chairman of Worthing Group Hospital Management Committee.
Jack A. Gilbey, Works Controller of Beecham Research Laboratories.
Harry T. Bunce, director of a Builders' Merchant Company.

Of this committee, Mrs. Lephard, Mr. Keeling and Mr. Bunce were all trustees of the Worthing Flower Fund.

Mr. B. Pennells was appointed architect to the committee.

Dr. Gusterson set out his own vision upon which the work of the committee would be firmly based:

Medical science is doing much to elucidate the problem of the cause, and hence to find the cure, of cancer. I doubt very much if this work is being held up by lack of money.

There still remains, and will for a long time to come, the plight of many people for whom there can be no curative treatment. This is a need which surely is a charge on the sympathy of everybody and is the challenge we are accepting at this new home.

Suffering, whether it be physical, mental or spiritual, is something which can only be dealt with by those with a great love for their fellows, and this is the work we are asking people to share in by supporting this new home.

Those who subsequently witnessed the dedication and work of 'Gus' himself will verify the full extent to which he met the standards he set out in that last paragraph.

The appeal committee held their meetings at the offices of the Worthing Hospital Management Committee and were allowed the part-time use of an office. Dr. Gusterson saw this as one sign of what he termed 'the very happy relationship with the Hospital Authorities from the very beginning'. A further sign was the understanding approach shown by the Regional Hospital Board when, at a very early stage, he and Dr. Franks had discussed the question of contractual beds. The helpful attitude of the Board was to prove vital in the early days of financial uncertainty as the Home began to care for its patients. Mrs. D. Alvey acted as part-time secretary to the appeal in the early days, a fact which led Dr. Gusterson to express his appreciation of not only her work but that of a host of volunteers who helped quietly and unostentatiously behind the scenes. At one stage they did consider hiring a professional fund-raiser but decided against on the basis that their appeal was to people's sympathy for and understanding of the needs of others, and that people would respond generously. They were correct.

The appeal for the Home was launched at a press conference at Beecham's Research Laboratories on Friday 20 October 1967. Some sobering statistics were read out, not least that cancer was the cause of almost 20 per cent of deaths in the Worthing area and that many died outside a hospital bed. This enabled Dr. Gusterson to stress that hospitals were 'essentially places for active treatment and curable diseases'. People in the last stages of illness needed devoted time from the nursing staff which 'with the best will in the world cannot always be done by nurses working in busy wards in general hospitals'. Those were the reasons why an appeal for £100,000 (over £800,000 at 1998 values) was being launched to build a home. The appeal was, he thought, probably the largest ever made in Worthing. It would have 30 to 40 beds with a high ratio of nurses to give devoted care. Spiritual care would be available when needed. A mixture of wards and individual rooms and adequate residential accommodation would be provided for nursing and other staff. In addition to the ward block there would be a chapel, an administrative section, lounges for patients and visitors and rooms for relatives. Apart from resident patients, some would be admitted for short stays to relieve relatives from nursing care so they could go on holiday.

The home would be non-profit making. Charges for patients would depend on how much money was raised before the home was opened. Many patients would not be able to afford the full maintenance cost, so it was hoped that charitable funds would be available to ensure that no patient was refused admission because of inability to pay.

It had been decided to name the home St Barnabas'. This came about when, at the end of the first meeting of the committee, Mrs. Lephard asked: 'What are we going to call this home? We must think of something nicer than "Terminal Home for cancer patients"'. Canon Reeves was asked if he could suggest a suitable saint. Next morning, after looking up his reference books, he rang Dr. Gusterson: 'It is the Eve of the Feast of St Barnabas today. He was the Saint of Consolation, you know'. Dr. Gusterson didn't – but realised that the choice of the name was inspired.

St Barnabas was a rich young Jewish Cypriot, a contemporary of St Paul, who sold all his lands and gave the money to the church in Antioch when they were in great need. His name was Joseph but the apostles named him Barnabas, meaning 'Son of Consolation'. He had a strong interest in people. A phrase in the Acts of the Apostles describes him as 'a good man full of the Holy Spirit, and of faith'. Thus the appeal became known as The St Barnabas' Appeal.

Just after this decision was made, Dr. Gusterson met Mr. Charles Hunnibal of Lancing and asked him to design a suitable motif for the Appeal. The design, still in use today, shows St Barnabas holding the Bible in one hand and in the other, outstretched in blessing, are shells of edible shellfish of the Mediterranean Sea, the traditional symbol of the traveller.

The appeal to raise the £100,000 was officially launched at a public meeting in the Assembly Hall on Friday 29 March 1968. The *Worthing Gazette* remarked that the day after the Budget was probably not the best time to think about giving money away, but about 250 came to the meeting. The speaker was Dr. Cicely Saunders who founded the St Christopher's Hospice in Sydenham.

Dr. Saunders was the leading authority on the scope of homes for the terminally ill. Her own idea to establish a home came to her after talking to a patient with advanced cancer. 'He needed friendship and an opportunity to look back on his life so that he could finish it in fullness and not emptiness. When he died he left me £500 to start the work.' (Her life's work is described in Shirley de Boulay's book, *Cicely Saunders, The Founder of the Modern Hospice Movement*, published by Hodder and Stoughton.) She set out the aims of such homes as to help relieve suffering and provide real friendship so that patients could find inner peace. She showed slides of the £½ million London home which was helping people to cope with the overwhelming problems of incurable illness.

Her talk fired much enthusiasm for the project. The Archdeacon of Chichester, the Ven. Lancelot Mason, called the project, rather quaintly, 'Not only a must – it is a mustest'. He was particularly interested because it would provide an outlet for voluntary service. Similar views were expressed by Monsignor A.C. Iggleden, the Roman Catholic priest of Worthing, and the Revd. Hubert Janisch.

Dr. Gusterson would dearly have liked to announce the site of the new home but, as he put it, 'there are some difficulties over negotiations'. (Anyone who knew Dr. Gusterson will vouch for his ability to express in simple, understated sentences situations which were complex and difficult to unravel.) He was able to report, however, that £4,500 had already been raised.

To list the contributors to the fund would be tedious but some examples will suffice to show the kind of response. One anonymous donor offered to contribute £1,000 (£8,000 at 1998 values) provided that within six months another five donors would do likewise, or ten would donate £500 each. Only one other donor responded so the offer was withdrawn. However, contributions came in steadily, usually in small amounts, sometimes as the result of special fund-raising efforts. For example, £100 was donated by the Worthing and District Ladies Auxiliary League of the Licensed Victuallers Association. A grant of £1,000 was received from the West Sussex County Council. At a tea party held by The Priory, which he had helped to found, Dr. Gusterson was presented with a cheque for £25 to thank him for the security which he had given to the residents. Although most donations were small, by early 1968 they were totalling £50 to £100 a week; by June, when the total was £15,000, there had been over 600 individual donations.

In 1968, the committee invited the Duke of Norfolk to be their President. His response was enthusiastic, and together with the Duchess he was to show a lively interest in the life of the Home, often making informal visits. In the same year, St Barnabas' was registered as a charity.

It was perhaps inevitable that not everyone would give their support to the appeal, or even the concept of a home for the terminally ill. In the middle of 1968, the

Honorary Secretary of the West Sussex Nursing Homes Association, Mr. Edgar Gisby, wrote to the *Worthing Herald* criticising the plans to build a home for the terminally sick. 'We support the St Barnabas' appeal for funds but we feel that a special building will swallow up too much money.' With more contractual beds in nursing homes, catering for the same type of cases, the appeal fund would be better used in helping 'the penurious sick' with fees for those beds. 'St Barnabas' will not be ready for three years and the need is here and urgent now.'

He returned to the offensive in March 1969, claiming that patients entering St Barnabas' would be charged up to 25gns a week. He estimated that from interest on the £46,000 raised at that time, nine people could be kept in a nursing home for a whole year. The proprietors of the homes had £1 million invested in the town and had all the facilities to offer. He wrote to each member of the St Barnabas' committee inviting them to 'reconsider the whole project before committing themselves to purchasing the site'.

Dr. Gusterson strongly refuted these claims. Although a charge of 20-25gns would be made, 'those who genuinely could not afford it would not have to pay that sum. There would be organisations helping by raising money to provide beds for these people. We will definitely never turn away people because they have insufficient money'.

He found it 'distressing' to 'have to deal with someone at cross purposes when dealing with humanitarian works'. He robustly rejected Mr. Gisby's request for a public meeting so that those who had given money so far could decide 'what they would rather do with their money'.

The next month Mr. Gisby had cause to celebrate. The South-West Metropolitan Hospital Board announced that it had allocated £20,000 per year for the next four or five years to enable contracts to be made with selected nursing homes to take geriatric patients from the hospitals in the area. Mr. Gisby commented that with these developments the St Barnabas' Home 'could be used for the poorest sick without having to charge them fees, so that it would become a true charity'.

Dr. Gusterson was not someone to be mealy-mouthed where important matters were at stake. In May 1969 he addressed the Worthing Committee of the National Society for Cancer Research. In describing the purpose-built facilities which were to be provided, with plenty of space and light with 'gracious nurses' tending to their needs and with loneliness now having no meaning, he compared that vision with 'current practices'. These included, he said,

> many patients ... having to live three in a room on top of a third floor attic, with a constant smell of stale urine to remind them of their plight. Somebody has got to say it ... and it is going on. These places must be made unnecessary, redundant.

Not surprisingly, these remarks brought a reaction – from the West Sussex Nursing Homes Association, although Mr. Gisby had now been succeeded by Mr. Norman Evans. He refuted the claims made by Dr. Gusterson; such conditions 'would not be tolerated by the County Council nursing homes inspector' who made unscheduled three-monthly visits, and he maintained that the allegations were slanderous. He accused him of a sanctimonious 'holier than thou' attitude; he challenged the doctor to name names publicly or else provide the medical officer of health in Chichester with the details. He also attacked Dr. Gusterson's phrase 'gracious nurses'; Swandean Hospital had recently closed eight beds because of a nursing shortage – 'where is the good doctor going to find the surfeit of gracious nurses out of the hat'?

The 'good doctor' was away on holiday when these accusations were made but Mr. Joseph Sayers came to his defence. In some nursing homes the accommodation was not what it should be, but there were nevertheless some very good homes in the cheaper price bracket. A large number were run extremely well but there were others which left a lot to be desired. In his opinion, the attention which patients would receive at St Barnabas' would be 'second to none'; those types of homes always attracted the nurse who was 'really dedicated to caring for such people'.

Whatever the motivation of those who had objections to the concept of the Home, it is fair to say that the great majority of Worthing residents realised how much St Barnabas' would have to offer, and they saw to it by their continuing support that Dr. Gusterson's vision would become reality.

The original idea of the committee was to build the home in Worthing with easy access to public transport, but the acqusition of a suitable site proved to be a major headache. Although several possibilities were discussed with the Town Council, ranging from Shelley Road to the 18th tee of the Worthing Golf Course, there were always significant drawbacks.

In December 1968 the finance and law committee of the Worthing Town Council recommended that corporation land at Titnore Lane, on the north side of Upper Northbrook Farm Lane near the corporation's new nurseries, should be provided. A 60-year lease was proposed.

The encouraging response from the Council was enough for the committee to put the following advertisement in the *Worthing Herald* on 14 March 1969:

ST. BARNABAS HOME

STOP PRESS NEWS!

SITE:
Thanks to the co-operation of the Worthing Town Council we have been offered a two acre site in the Titnore Road area at an economic rent. This has enabled us to go right ahead with the Architect's plans. Subject to Planning Permission it is hoped that building will start during 1969.

FINANCE:
At least £100,000 is required. Of this we have already received £45,000. This leaves £55,000 urgently required, which in fact means less than Ten Shillings from each member of the population of the Worthing Hospital Group Area.

Information from 1 St. George's Road, Worthing

2   Worthing Herald *appeal, 1969*

In April 1969 the West Sussex County Council directed the Town Council to reject the application. They ruled that the site was too far out of town in a place where there was not adequate transport. It would also mean a departure from the development plan which classified it as 'white land'. Dr. Gusterson was disappointed; however, he could see that the site, although quiet and ideal for patients in the last stages of illness, would have been largely inaccessible for domiciliary staff. He bravely declared it to be a 'temporary setback' although the frustration generated by the process was such that by now he had almost thrown in the towel.

As something of a last attempt, it was decided to make an approach direct to the West Sussex County Council and a meeting was held in County Hall, Chichester of which the eventual outcome was that the County suggested a site which they owned in Columbia Drive, west of Durrington Lane. (Columbia Drive was named in memory of the Canadians who were stationed in the Durrington area during the war.) The Worthing Town Council planning committee was ready to give outline planning permission for the site, and leave the County planning committee to endorse their approval, as well as to negotiate terms for the lease or sale of the land. The cost of the land was £30,000 and the County Council gave a two-year period of grace for the sum to be repaid.

Dr. Gusterson professed himself satisfied. The site was indeed much more accessible and had the advantage of being within a growing community. The *Worthing Gazette*'s photograph of Dr. Gusterson standing in the ploughed field, visualising the building, is a vivid record of someone who had stuck valiantly to his task and who could now see his vision about to take shape in tangible bricks and mortar.

With this rosier prospect in view, the practical elements of the project were initiated. The plans which had been on hold for so long were now dusted down and revised in detail. Drawing, re-drawing and all manner of amendments were now the order of the day, with the architect, Mr. Bernard Pennells, and his team now being able to get their teeth into the project after many years of waiting and uncertainty.

Then came another show-stopper. The result of trial boreholes showed that the water table was only 3ft. 6in. below the surface. Water drained off the chalk hills onto the clay at Durrington and ponds quickly formed in wet weather. To erect a two-storey building, as envisaged, on foundations of such 'crust thickness' would require the construction of 30-foot piles to support it.

This could quadruple the cost, and the committee paled at the thought of a £400,000 target (over £3 million at today's values).

An alternative design was then proposed: a single-storey construction using prefabricated units. Not only would this avoid the cost of piling, and shorten the building time, but being single-storey would eliminate the expensive lifts which the original plan envisaged. By September 1970 the committee agreed to proceed, estimating the cost of the building to be £60,000 and access roads and drains etc. £35,000.

The committee now had to face up to the financial situation. By the end of April 1971 the total raised had reached £76,000, the inflow of donations having improved dramatically since the permission to build had been given.

There was, however, still a shortfall of £30,000. They decided to approach the National Society for Cancer Relief which had just launched an appeal for £1 million to build ten such homes in memory of the Olympic athlete, Lillian Board. Dr. Gusterson,

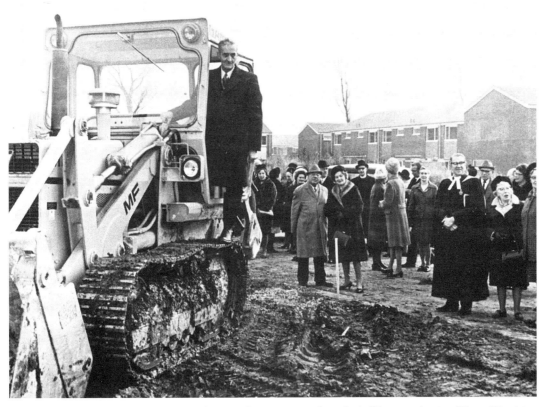

3   *The Mayor of Worthing, Alderman Sydney Knight, prepares to drive the bulldozer on the site. (Photo:* Worthing Herald*)*

Mr. Bunce and Mr. Keeling attended a meeting of the Society's Council in July. Privately, they were sure that the Society would not be able to meet such an ambitious building programme for that amount of money, and they suggested that St Barnabas' might be included in the Society's scheme. This suggestion was not taken up but they were listened to sympathetically and in August received a donation of £10,000. The Society said that it was not their normal policy to make capital grants for buildings but they had been impressed by the efforts which had been made to raise so much capital. They would still be interested in supporting St Barnabas' when the patients began to be admitted.

Meanwhile, there had been another significant event. Dr. Gusterson relates it thus in his history:

> On June 11, 1971 (St Barnabas' Day), I attended an early Service at a small country Church. Only the Rector and myself were present. We both had in mind the great need of the Home. That afternoon I was telephoned by a Worthing Solicitor to tell me that he had a client who would like to loan the St Barnabas' Home £25,000 free of interest. The donor wished to remain anonymous but the loan was to 'enable us to get the building started'. I tell this story without further comment and leave you to make your own.

This was a great boost to the morale of the committee which, at times, had felt despondent. Tenders were now sent out to seven local firms in early October. The date for opening the returned bids was 9 November 1971. The lowest was for £111,061 by Messrs B. Cheal & Sons. This was accepted by the committee. Work was to begin on 8 December 1971 with a contract time of 52 weeks.

The cost of the total project, however, including the land, was now about £180,000. The committee expected to incur a bank overdraft although the Treasurer, Mr. Burnham Roe, thought that the bank might well be prepared to cover it without any charge of interest. In the event, no such overdraft became necessary.

Dr. Gusterson describes the ceremony to begin the work on the site:

> The actual commencement of the building was marked by a somewhat unusual ceremony. Owing to the construction of the building an ordinary stone-laying ceremony was not possible. We therefore invited the then mayor, Councillor S. Knight, to drive the first bulldozer in the presence of invited guests. As it was then the middle of winter, we could not have long outdoor speeches. The Temperance Building Society offered us the hospitality of their Conference Room, where the speeches were made. We then moved to the site where prayers of thanksgiving and blessing were said by Canon J.W. Reeves and the Rev. H. Janisch.

In spite of having to concentrate on these difficulties, the committee had not ignored other matters needing their attention. A sub-committee was briefed to ensure that the necessary fitting up and provision of equipment was in place by completion. In January 1969 two senior sisters from Worthing Hospital, Miss Frieda Sackse and Miss Irene Nelson, expressed a wish to help and were invited to advise on planning and equipment. During one whole weekend, Miss Sackse with the Matron of Southlands Hospital, Miss Pilbeam, produced a 'room loading schedule' which set out in detail every item of furniture and equipment required in each room.

As early as February 1971 Dr. Gusterson could claim that he had six nursing staff waiting to take up appointments as soon as the home was built. He also emphasised that many of those who would help at the home would be doing so on a voluntary basis – 'people who really want to help others' – and their dedication would enrich the feeling of care in the home. In July 1972 it was announced that Dr. Gusterson had been appointed medical director, with Dr. R.E. Francis as medical consultant. The appointment of Matron was given to Miss Sackse and the post of senior nursing sister to Miss Nelson, formerly a theatre sister at Worthing Hospital. Miss Sackse regarded her appointment 'as a very great honour'. She had begun her training at Hemel Hempstead, did midwifery at Eastbourne (her home town) followed by further training at Bournemouth. At the beginning of the war she was at the Nelson Hospital in Wimbledon. She went to India with the Queen Alexandra Imperial Nursing Service Reserve and was matron at a hospital on the North West frontier. Psychiatric nursing at Roffey Park Hospital, Faygate followed before being appointed assistant matron at Newton Abbot. She spent nine years as administrative sister at Worthing and then four years as assistant matron. Her decision to offer her services to the home, in spite of her real enjoyment in attending her garden at her Lancing home after retirement, meant that the staff were guided by someone with extensive experience and someone who, as she put it, had 'always liked people'.

Dr. Gusterson made an appeal 'for one or two very good cooks because we are anxious that the food served to patients at our new home will be of the highest standard'; food from the kitchen would be taken in a heated cabinet straight to the bedside.

Meanwhile, the construction was going ahead, with Mr. Harry Bunce, chairman of the building sub-committee, keeping a very watchful eye on the contractors. He had used his expertise to purchase expensive items early; the only significant inflationary cost to the project was a wage rise for some of the construction workers amounting to an extra £3,000.

In September 1972, Dr. Gusterson was able to boast that they had almost enough nursing staff 'without any advertising'. Some minor grades were still needed, and a cook, but they had sufficient staff to admit 12 patients. Although the building fund was still short of £42,000 he considered that they had done 'unbelievably well'. He said that as soon as the building costs were paid for, legacies would be used to build up an endowment fund to help those patients who could not find the full maintenance costs themselves. The Regional Hospital Board had agreed in principle to contractual arrangements for some of the beds, which meant that quite a few of them would be paid for entirely by the Board. But, he added, 'the days of miracles are not yet ended. There are still the miracles of human compassion, sympathy and understanding'.

Some introductory tours of the buildings were held. On one such occasion, the presentation of a cheque for £1,000 from the West Sussex Travel Society was made. A press photograph bears a long caption with a striking conclusion; it describes how

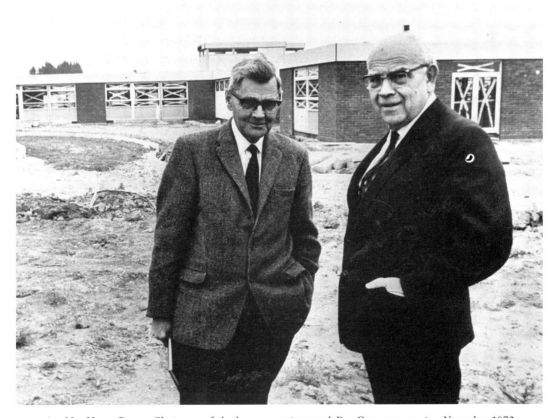

4 *Mr. Harry Bunce, Chairman of the house committee and Dr. Gusterson on site, November 1972*

the party admired 'the wide doorways to all the rooms which allow beds to be wheeled from ward to ward, or ward to washroom, in which patients will be lifted from beds by special hoist and hosed down shower fashion'(!).

Dr. Gusterson wrote in his history:

> We took possession of the building on December 7th according to the Contract, though as usual there were many finishing touches required. In fact the first few weeks of December were the scene of many hectic activities, our nursing staff and stewards, members of the Committee and volunteers from the St John's Ambulance Brigade, all moving in equipment or cleaning.

Amongst the staff were Peter Hutchinson and Peter Lock who were formerly theatre technicians at Worthing Hospital; they were titled stewards at St Barnabas'. Their role was to care for the patients in the morning and in the afternoon to turn their hand to any task that might need attention, although any patient need would take priority. Among their unpredictable duties, they painted the old iron beds which had been acquired from the hospital, cleared out concrete from the drains which the builders' work generated and chased away gypsies' ponies that would stray into the vegetable patch! These tasks were cheerfully carried out because Dr. Gusterson was a man whose enthusiasm was infectious, as was his high energy level. He and his wife camped in the building for several days at the end of December for security reasons, Dorothy preparing their meals in the kitchen and their family joining them from time to time.

The dedication service of St Barnabas' was held at 10.30am on Friday 29 December 1972, led by the Rt. Revd. Evered Lunt representing the Lord Bishop of Chichester. Each significant room was blessed, including the Day Room where the altar was placed and where the final act of dedication was made. The choir of St Paul's Church sang the anthem 'If ye love me, keep my commandments', the Collect for St Barnabas was read before the blessing, and the service ended with the choir singing 'God be in my head'. The following day the Home, with its two 12-bedded wards and six single rooms, and with a trained staff of 20, was open to the public from 10am to 6pm and over 2,000 people visited. The first patients were admitted the next day, Monday 1 January 1973.

Shortly afterwards, the Chairman of the St Barnabas' Council, Mr. Burnham Roe (the former Treasurer), paid tribute to Dr. Gusterson

> whose dedication and leadership brought this work to fruition. Ever since the first meeting of the steering committee on the Eve of St Barnabas in June, 1967 Dr. Gusterson has never failed to take the chair at the monthly meetings.

He also paid tribute to Mr. Harry Bunce for the weeks he had spent 'planning, selecting, ordering and receiving the 1001 pieces of necessary equipment'. All this, he said, had grown from the first donation, which was of 10 shillings in September 1967.

CHAPTER 2

THE CARING BEGINS

The response from the Worthing area and beyond, from groups and individuals alike, had at first grown quietly and steadily. Some examples will suffice, although they are only the tip of the iceberg.

In September 1968 an anonymous gift of £1,000 was received from Sidmouth in Devon. To ensure that the donor's identity would not be revealed, the gift was prepared in the form of a cheque signed by a bank manager.

On 29 September 1968 a sponsored walk took place from Worthing to Hove and back, co-ordinated by Mr. Duncan McNeil, chairman of the appeals liaison committee, and staff nurse Sandra Bower of Worthing Hospital. Nearly 150 took part, but those to catch the eye were a team of nurses from the hospital who hitched their uniform skirts eight inches above the knee for the occasion! 'We are getting some new uniforms soon, but I can't see the skirts getting quite this high', commented one of the girls. Also sponsored was Rex, an Alsatian dog, at over £1 a mile. The first to complete the 25-mile route, in 4hr 35min, was Mr. R.L. Hutchinson of Beechams, who was welcomed home by Dr. Gusterson with a promised bottle of champagne. The walk raised over £500.

Also in September, Beecham Research Laboratories handed over a cheque for £750. Many of their employees took part in the charity walk, but Dr. Gusterson welcomed the donation as 'the first contribution to the fund from local business. We hope that other local firms will feel that they can also help in this way'. This was a hope that was more than fulfilled as the years passed, and local businesses were to play an important part in providing finance, goods and expertise.

The autumn of 1968 saw many contributions from local churches and organisations; for example, St John's Church, Worthing gave £41, the Worthing Mayflower Club £36, the Worthing Ladies Circle £65 and the Durrington Townswomen's Guild 30gns.

This all prompted Dr. Gusterson to write a letter to the *Worthing Herald* just before Christmas in which he expressed 'the hope that all who have helped us may themselves find real happiness at Christmas time'. He felt that the attraction of the appeal was summed up by two donations he had recently received – one an anonymous donation of £2,000, the other four shillings in cash from a blind pensioner.

One rather unsavoury event caused him to write to the *Gazette* in August 1969:

> It has been brought to my notice that people are being called upon in their homes and asked to subscribe to the St Barnabas' Appeal. I have no knowledge of any such action, which would certainly not be approved of by the Appeal Committee. All those working for the appeal carry official recognition notes, and I would ask anyone who is approached by someone they do not know to ask for a sight of this note.

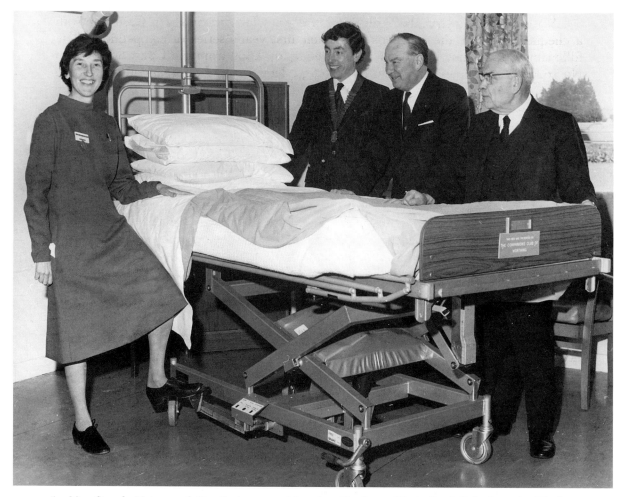

5   *Miss Stroud, Matron and Dr. Gusterson receiving the gift of two King's Fund Beds from the Worthing Companions Club, with Mr. John Wright, Chairman and Mr. Harry Dobson. (Photo:* Evening Argus*)*

In 1969 the profits from the production of 'Boeing-Boeing' by the West Sussex Players in The Pavilion, Worthing from 5-8 February, were given to the appeal; the same happened at a military band concert in August given by the Band of H.M. Royal Marines, and with a Sunday evening concert given by the Central Band of the Women's Royal Air Force in October.

One local resident, Mrs. M. Maskell, who had been confined to a wheelchair for two years, decided to run her own 'small sale' at her home in St Thomas' Road. She wrote to each person in the road inviting them to her bungalow. On the morning of her sale, having herself spent weeks making calendars, cards and toothbrush holders, people brought scarves, preserves, home-made cakes, toys and toiletries. Mrs. Maskell raised nearly £22.

However, as soon as permission to build the Home was received, the rate of contributions increased markedly; people were able to see that their donations were to be directed towards a tangible, achievable result.

The Caring Begins

At the end of the year, the Worthing Lions 200 Club presented Dr. Gusterson with a cheque for £750, the proceeds from their first year's series of competitions. The following January saw him receiving a cheque for £300 from the Court Sussex Elm No 162 of the Independent Order of Foresters. These and other organisations were to remain stalwart supporters of the appeal and of the Home.

An individual achievement in 1970 was that of Mr. Duncan McNeil (the organiser of the charity walk) who, at the age of 70, accomplished a 40-mile walk after having an arthritic hip replaced. His sponsorship card read: 'A lone walker will attempt the Sussex Downs Way walk from Eastbourne to Worthing during the week ending 25 September' and invited sponsorship at ½d., 1d. or 3d. per mile. He raised over £50 on the walk which lasted three days, spending two nights out camping.

Early in 1970, the Worthing Companions Club announced the formation of a fund to perpetuate the memory of their founder, Mr. Harold Frampton. He had founded the club in 1956 to assist 'people who [find] themselves in unexpected and unfortunate circumstances'. The club committee thought that a fitting way to honour him would be to provide a 'Harold Frampton Room' with furnishings and fittings, for the use of the patients and their relatives in the St Barnabas' Home. The aim was to raise £500. At the same time, the Worthing Inner Wheel promised to make itself financially responsible for the layout of the forecourt. This prompted Dr. Gusterson to say that his committee hoped that people would like the idea of having specific rooms or beds dedicated to the memory either of their friends or of societies and organisations, and he prepared a list of suitable sums for such purposes.

At the end of April 1971 the Treasurer of the appeal, Mr. Burnham Roe, at a meeting in the Richmond Room, received cheques totalling £862. This sum included contributions from the Worthing Soroptimists, the Companions Club, the Worthing Musical Comedy Society and, curiously, the Noel Buxton Trust, a charity originally set up to combat slavery. 'We hope that the St Barnabas' Home will relieve the slavery of fear' was Dr. Gusterson's highly appropriate response.

In May, in the Mayor's Parlour, a £250 cheque and a scroll with the names of those who contributed was presented by the West Nova Scotia Regiment. The 'West Novies' were stationed in and around Durrington during the Second World War. The donation was in appreciation of the many acts of kindness displayed towards the regiment. The money would be allocated towards the furnishing of a room in the Home.

One of the members of the appeal committee, addressing the West Chiltington Flower Club about the Home, was overwhelmed when someone present donated £5,000 on hearing about the need (a gift worth £40,000 at 1998 values).

Our final example concerns a source of income which has proved to be the lifeblood of St Barnabas' – legacies. Early in 1970, the fund received the considerable sum of £11,245 from the will of the late Mr. William Sloss, a former director of Lever Brothers, who lived in Cecilian Avenue. The value of legacies can hardly be overstated as the accounts of St Barnabas' have shown over its 25-year history.

One continuing group of supporters must be mentioned here – the congregation and parishioners of St Mary's Church, Thakeham, where Dr. Gusterson worshipped and later led the services as a Reader. They raised £350 at one coffee morning alone.

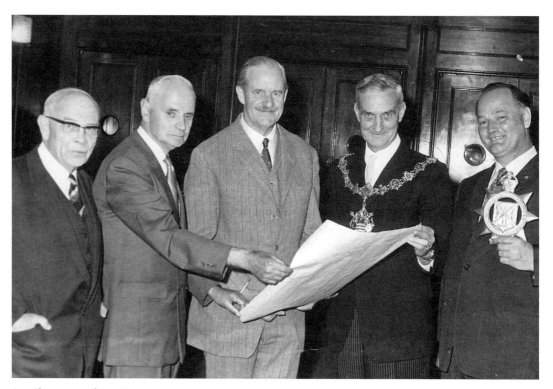

6 *The Mayor of Worthing receives a cheque from Major-General Pat Bogart (representing the Canadian High Commissioner) from the veterans of the West Nova Scotia Regiment, with Dr. Gusterson, Mr. Keith Clarke and Mr. Abbie Warlin of the Regiment. (Photo:* Worthing Herald*)*

In 1969, a festival of flowers with the theme 'Meditation on the Creed' raised £300. The following year the theme was 'Handel's Messiah' and the sum rose to over £400. The church was more than once the venue for thanksgiving services for St Barnabas'.

This was the background of local support which enabled the Home to open its doors and so began the first full operating year of 'St Barnabas' Nursing Home Ltd., Worthing', to give it its full title.

The 'Memorandum and Articles of Association' were the work of the legal adviser, Mr. Richard Stapleton, and set out the constitution of the Home. There were to be 20 members of the Association. Provision was made for an annual general meeting, voting rights etc. There was to be a Council of at least ten in number but the day-to-day running was administered by the House Committee, itself responsible to the Council. The chairman of this committee was elected annually, and the first chairman was Mr. H.T. Bunce. The Medical Director and the Matron had entire responsibility for the admission and nursing care of patients, who would only be admitted with their GP's approval and after a visit by the Medical Director.

The first admissions were at the rate of one or two at a time so that the necessary nursing routine could be properly established. Nine patients were admitted during the first two weeks of January 1973, of whom five died within that time. Whilst the build-up of the nursing staff proceeded satisfactorily, there was some difficulty in finding staff for the kitchen, especially for the evenings and weekends.

The fluid staff situation meant that the Bursar, Mr. Bradwell, was in the dark about the running costs, which for the first six weeks came to £1,300, including salaries. The Regional Hospital Board, which had agreed to fund eight beds at a daily rate of £6.85, had contracted to pay their grant quarterly in arrears, which did not assist cash flow. Income aside from this consisted of an average £8 per week from the collection box in the entrance hall; the first donations totalled £50 and donations in lieu of flowers £30. The bank balance was £10,000 of which half was earning interest. The costs for staff meals were fixed at 25p for lunch, 15p for supper, 15p for breakfast, coffee 5p and tea 3p.

The House Committee, at their meeting on 16 January 1973, attempted to establish the ground rules for their method of operating. Their order of priority makes interesting reading.

First, they tackled the handling of complaints from patients or relatives. These were to be made in writing and attended to immediately by the Chairman or, if he were absent, by another member of the committee after consultation with Dr. Gusterson. The chairman would report to the committee at its next meeting. Second, the committee had to approve all items of capital expenditure, referring larger amounts to the Council. The same applied to all staff appointments, except for the Medical Director, Matron and Bursar. Next, a procedure for ensuring that all patient costs were covered was to be set up and fifth, all patients' local – but not long distance – telephone calls could be made without charge, as any system of recording and collection would be out of all proportion to the sums involved.

They next decided that flowers should be financed from a designated account. The lady arrangers, supervised by Mrs. Bollom, could either negotiate with a local florist who would invoice the Bursar, or provide their own flowers if they so wished.

The necessary insurance of the buildings and equipment was taken out with the Sun Alliance at an annual premium of £1,359.

The question of locum cover was raised. It was agreed to go ahead so that Dr. Gusterson could take holidays and be covered for any absences through sickness. The minutes of the first meeting then state:

> Dr. Gusterson expressed his thanks for this kind gesture and stated that one of the first things he intended to do in view of his age, was to try to find a replacement, so that there would be adequate time to train his successor. This situation also applied to Matron, who had come out of retirement in order to get the Home organised and running smoothly.

It was felt that the Home was not yet in a sufficiently organised state to use volunteers, but a list was kept of those people who were offering their services.

Finally, all monies donated by the relatives of patients who had died at the Home were to be placed in a special fund kept by the Treasurer.

We shall see that questions concerning admission policy, relationships with local GPs, staffing levels, finance, links with the Health Authority and the role of visitors provide a constant theme around which the committee worked.

A month later, the committee were told that the Council did not agree with their proposals about capital expenditure but wished all such items to be referred to them. But the Council met less frequently, so its Chairman, Mr. Roe and its Treasurer, Mr. Davey could be consulted if there were a matter of urgency. In the meantime, further bids for insurance cover were being invited and the nurse call system was being extended. Dr. Gusterson reported that 41 patients had been admitted. Six of these had either gone home or were expected to do so shortly. This was a feature that he wanted to be publicised; it was one of his major worries that the public regarded the Home as a place of last resort to which a patient only went when death was the only expectation.

The Bursar was asked to be responsible for assessing the financial status of the patients. The principle of the Home was that care would be given regardless of anyone's financial situation. Treatment was free but from those who could afford to make a contribution, that was gratefully received.

The financial balancing act which was to exercise the members of the committee and the Council for many years was described very clearly in a report from the Bursar:

> We had admitted 41 patients, who had occupied 215 days in contractual beds, for which we shall receive £1,472 in fees: 166 days of fee paying patients had been used, for which we had received £882 and invoiced a further £272: 50 days of part paying and NSCR patients had been used, for which we had received £175 and invoiced a further £15. Several part weeks had not yet been invoiced. Out of 1,530 days of bed availability, we had used 475. In other words, we had only been one third full for 50 days since opening.

On the one hand, it was desirable to have as high a bed occupancy as possible, since the staffing levels were geared accordingly. Occupancy itself could be variable due to the nature of the patients' illnesses, whch required a varying level of treatment, some cases being much heavier than others; it was also impossible to predict the number of patients to be admitted. On the other hand, having established funding from the local health authority and the NSCR, there was every pressure to ensure that their funds were spent in line with their contracts. If funded beds were lying empty, the funding itself was threatened. Additionally, where patients were able to make a contribution to their nursing costs, such income was most welcome, indeed essential, but could not be guaranteed. Any shortfall in patient numbers had an inevitable impact on income whilst expenses remained the same.

Each bed cost £55 per day, wages and salary costs representing 73 per cent of that amount.

A comment in the Minutes records that 'food costs are most reasonable and our Cook is worth several hundred pounds a year in the economy and buying expertise she practises, besides giving patients and staff really enjoyable meals'.

Dr. Gusterson reported on the experiences of patient admission and care. There had been a very rapid turnover of cases and particular difficulty had been experienced with short-stay cases. This was due to the fact that their relatives had not been adequately prepared for what was going on in the Home and would not accept that their loved ones were dying. He was having to spend a lot of time with them to prepare them for the inevitable. He felt that some doctors had not at first appreciated the service the Home offered, although there had now been 36 referrals from GPs.

It was decided not to admit geriatric patients. Not only was this outside the responsibility of the Home but it was not right to place patients in the company of geriatrics, 'as the former needed a happy, cheerful and peaceful atmosphere in which to end their days'.

Meanwhile, the grounds were benefiting from the attention of Mr. Jack Watts, whose contribution to the gardens was to be long-lasting. The ploughing, hoeing and grass seeding had cost £250. There were ample funds to pay for the purchase of trees and plants. Seedlings were already being raised in boxes to be ready both for planting in due course and to provide cut flowers for decorating the home. A quotation was accepted for garden maintenance at £250 plus mowing at £1 per time. However, this did not include weeding the flower beds, and it was hoped that this would be done by Mr. Withers, one of the stewards. Plants for the centre bed, provided by Messrs A. Goatcher & Son cost £149.77, most of which was covered by donations.

On 1 March 1973 three visitors from Northampton, who were considering establishing a similar home, were extremely impressed by what they saw, and left with the intention of producing a replica of St Barnabas'. This was only the beginning of a series of visits from all over the United Kingdom, plus many from overseas. The Home was to become a centre with its own high reputation serving as a model for other bodies wishing to set up similar facilities. St Barnabas' was the third such Home to be built (after homes in Sheffield and Manchester).

At this time, an appeal was made for volunteers to help serve teas to patients and visitors. One of the first to respond was the Amberley Young Wives Group known as 'The Ladybirds' and whose founder was the wife of the vicar of Amberley. They did submit a request for some help with petrol costs. The committee's reply was that, as a charity, they had no authority to pay for petrol and with the increasing number of volunteers, to do so would lead rapidly to an escalation of costs.

One unpleasant incident occurred in March. A set of tools, valued at £40-£50, was stolen from one of the garages where staff bicycles were parked. With a change of insurer pending, it was thought appropriate to make a speedy claim on Sun Alliance. The police were notified and took plaster casts of a set of footprints found in the field outside the fence.

The Official Opening Ceremony was held on Monday, 18 June 1973 under the patronage of the Duchess of Roxburghe, chairman of the National Society for Cancer Relief (N.S.C.R.). Owing to a very crowded diary, the Duchess arrived by helicopter, touching down in the grounds of the nearby offices of the Temperance Building Society. She was welcomed by its General Manager, Mr. Sydney Burton and members of his staff, who had all been following the progress of the building programme over the past months from their vantage point in their multi-storey HQ, as well as making some financial donations to St Barnabas'. Although the Duchess slipped as she came down the steps from the helicopter, she was unhurt and went on to be welcomed by Dr. Gusterson and to address the 150 people at the ceremony, which was attended by representatives of local hospitals and organisations and two helpers from St Christopher's Hospice, Sydenham. She told them about the work of the Society, founded in the 1920's and which was at that time caring for about 11,000 patients. She unveiled a plaque, declared the Home open, toured the Home and met some of the patients and then had tea with the staff.

Dr. Gusterson and the Matron were invited to attend a conference called by St Christopher's Hospice, who were interested to know how St Barnabas' were faring; it seemed likely that they could well become the pattern for the smaller type of terminal home.

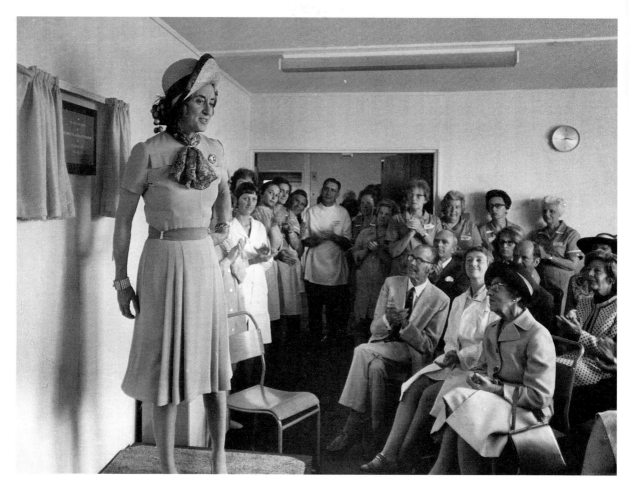
7   The Duchess of Roxburghe officially opens the St Barnabas' Nursing Home

   The problem of sources of referral continued. The majority of referrals were coming from medical social workers and health visitors rather than GPs who, it was felt, did not seem to appreciate when families were reaching the end of their tether. When they virtually collapsed from the strain of caring for a very ill relative, and only then, did the doctor request immediate admission as an emergency. One of the concerns that Dr. Gusterson had heard about was to learn from a patient's wife that, when patients were coming to St Barnabas', 'they had to be told they had cancer'. He asked all committee members 'to kill this rumour if ever they heard it mentioned'. The Home was to be described as one for 'people who were seriously ill and who needed special nursing care now, and we did not use the description "terminal home"'.

   The Bursar had to point out to the committee the impact of a national salary award recently made to nurses. It amounted to £1 per week plus 4 per cent of salary backdated. The cost, which had not been budgeted, would be an extra £50 per week. This would raise the bed cost by £1.50. He wanted the Regional Hospital Board to pay a higher rate for their contractual beds.

Dr. Gusterson raised the question of whether transport could be provided for patients' relatives, particularly those living outside the Worthing area who were without their own cars. The committee seized on this idea and also thought that they should set up a rota of drivers who could occasionally take patients out for drives. It was also important to involve as many people as possible in the work of St Barnabas'.

On 10 June a Thanksgiving Service for St Barnabas' Home was held at Thakeham Church, to which members of the staff, the Council and the House Committee were invited. Thakeham featured strongly in the loyal support of St Barnabas' over many years.

In May, Dr. Gusterson reported to the committee a sudden increase in admissions, so that there was now a waiting list. Of the 30 beds planned, two were still awaited from the manufacturer and two were always held free for possible emergency admissions. One of the difficulties was the contractual beds, numbering eight, for which the Regional Hospital Board paid. In order that this number could be honoured continually, it was necessary to have patients in the Home who could be transferred to these beds when they became vacant. Patients had been admitted even though the eight contractual beds were taken because it seemed wrong to have beds idle even though the Home did not receive a steady income from them. Hopefully, the contractual beds could be increased to ten. As the Bursar pointed out, the cost of not having more contractual beds was about £250 per week. Those who had to fund themselves could not hope to pay the full cost of £30 per week, and even those who were funded often could not reach the full cost. The Chairman of the House Committee, Mr. Bunce, felt that, even if the Home ran at a loss for the first year, it would nevertheless be achieving its aims.

Both he and Matron had noticed how the condition of some patients had improved dramatically after they had been at the Home for a few days. One patient had been able to return to her own home to end her days, as the staff had been able to prepare her and her family for this, and she knew that if necessary she could come back to St Barnabas'. Dr. Gusterson felt that this dramatic change in patients could 'only be due to the peace and quiet and excellent nursing care' the Home offered and it was therefore fulfilling what it had set out to do. He asked committee members to publicise the fact that patients did get better though their basic condition would still be there and they might need to return later on. Significantly, the Chairman and the committee stated that Dr. Gusterson and the Matron were to be congratulated for they themselves had created that atmosphere. One problem which could affect the number of admissions was the shortage of kitchen staff. The nurses had been helping as a temporary measure but could not do so indefinitely.

In his report to the committee on 19 June, Dr. Gusterson said that he had been told by the Duchess of Roxburghe that some hospitals were considering building terminal wings or buildings in their hospital grounds. He felt that this was a totally misconceived idea. The ideal situation was for a location quite separate from a hospital. Peace and quiet and a high staffing ratio was necessary and a small unit was preferable to a large one so that all the staff might become involved with the general care and welfare of the patients.

At this time, the final certificate for the building was issued by the architects together with the release of all the retentions. The final cost, including land, fixtures, fittings and equipment was £183,107, all paid for without needing any loan or overdraft.

A purpose-made Remembrance Book was placed in the Ante Room to record the names of all the patients who had died in the Home. The entries were to be handwritten by different members of the staff to make the entries more personal.

In June, the first issue of a Newsletter was in the last stages of preparation to be sent to 'our 2,000 odd subscribers'(!). The aim was to keep them in touch and to let them know of how donations had been spent and of current needs.

In July, the patients and staff were able to watch the Royal Wedding of Princess Anne and Capt. Mark Phillips on the colour television set in the Day Room. They all wore buttonholes and drank the health of the Royal couple as they emerged from the vestry after signing the register. Some patients sat through the whole service, having their lunches where they sat. At the end, one patient, who had never made a speech in her life, rose to say 'thank you' to the Matron and staff. Those who did not feel well enough to go into the Day Room were able to watch on the black and white sets in the wards. This included one patient who, although well enough to go into the Day Room, decided to stay in the ward with a friend who was not very well that day.

One unexpected and unwelcome event occurred on 11 August when Dr. Gusterson was taken ill very suddenly and rushed into Worthing Hospital. Dr. Kay, Assistant Medical Director, was away on holiday; Matron, Miss Sackse, who was also away for the same reason, was able to return at short notice and arrange for a doctor to be in the Home daily. She ensured that the Home continued to run on the pattern which Dr. Gusterson had set up.

She also made the home visits during this time. Dr. Gusterson sent a taped message expressing the hope that he would be able to resume light duties in about a month and expressing his pride in the way in which all the staff had carried on in his absence. In fact, he returned to duty on 15 October.

By this time, the number of contractual beds had been increased to 12, and the Bursar reported that bed occupancy had been 64 per cent, although it had reached 89 per cent for the past three months. The funding situation could best be described as uncertain. There was a shortage of regular income. The guaranteed income was £900 per week compared with outgoings of £1,550 per week. The Appeals Committee had just given him £5,500 and the weekly donations in lieu of flowers amounted to about £50. A sum of £500 was expected from the Friends of Worthing Hospitals for use in helping their former patients with their fees. £1,000 was outstanding from deceased patients' estates and another £1,000 from patients themselves. £800 from the next expected grant from the NSCR had already been used.

Not for the first – or last – time was the question of fees reviewed. The wording of the minutes of 16 October shows how carefully the balance was maintained:

> It was likely in some cases, we were not getting our due money from patients, as we had to accept their word on what savings and income they had: we could not talk to some patients about 'claiming on their estates', if they were unaware that their days were numbered: we should be careful never to agree to accept a set lower fee from patients in full settlement of their financial obligation to us, as this would legally preclude us from claiming on their estate.

As part of the publicity drive, it was decided to issue a brochure, using a donation of £1,000. It was planned 'to last indefinitely' and would therefore not include names of officials and staff. A loose slip would give details of fees and on the back of this would be given details of deeds of covenant, legacies and the exact title of the Home. The text itself required some careful study.

By the end of the year, Dr. Gusterson felt that 'the tension had gone out of the job now'. He said that all the staff were tired but the anxiety had gone and things were now running smoothly. This was supported by Matron.

There had been two complaints about the way patients were being handled. One concerned a case that had to be transferred to Graylingwell. The other involved someone who was unhappy about a friend's treatment. Dr. Gusterson investigated this case. He discovered that the patient had not accepted the true nature and inevitable outcome of her illness and had been resentful 'of everything and everybody'. Thus she had made unreasonable complaints against those who had tried to help her. Dr. Gusterson stressed that any little complaint should be taken up as a matter of policy.

On the financial side, as the end of the year approached, Mr. Bradwell was quoted as saying that, for the first time in almost nine months, he was 'happy about the financial position of the Home'. Total income for the first financial year was £107,475; the Hospital Board contribution was £27,198, the NSCR's £6,000 and patients' fees £27,901 with legacies totalling £26,299. Expenditure was £82,238 leaving an operating surplus of £25,237.

A full Christmas programme was organised. Four patients were able to return to their homes. Despite the fact that many of the remaining patients were very ill, they were all able to join in the festivities. The visit of the Mayor and Mayoress was a great success. All patients received a present, a glass of wine and a carnation buttonhole. The Night Staff held a party on 13 December, enabling them to meet many of the committee members.

The Day Staff had a party on 4 January which turned out to be 'a fantastic event'. Dr. Gusterson 'was so pleased that the old hospital tradition of holding a staff party had been revived at St Barnabas' and that Christmas had been an occasion of real joy and fun for everyone connected with the Home'.

As the first year ended, Dr. Gusterson announced that the new year would begin with a Communion Service celebrated by Bishop Lunt, in which some of the prayers from the Dedication Service would be said. He felt that this would be an appropriate occasion 'to re-dedicate ourselves to the particular type of work being carried out at St Barnabas' Home'. Its subsequent history is a sign of the extent and depth of that dedication.

CHAPTER 3
THE MISSION

Dr. Gusterson had claimed before the Home was built that it would be staffed by 'gracious nurses'. The nurses who joined the staff did so either because they knew him and his work (he was a charismatic character who was known to ask: 'Are you with me?') or because they were attracted by the style of nursing which was required. The latter meant 'bedside nursing', giving what is nowadays referred to as 'tender, loving care'. Gone was the conveyor-belt pressure of a main hospital ward and the need to move quickly to the next urgent task. With a ratio of 1.75 nurses to each bed, here was the opportunity to get to know each patient, and their family. Most of the nursing staff tended to be in their 40's or above, delighted to return to the basic nursing in which they had been trained. Some even came to St Barnabas' at a lower grade in order to achieve this high job satisfaction. Staff turnover was therefore relatively low. All of them had a great respect for Dr. Gusterson.

Nevertheless the arrival of the first patients had been a taxing time. Most of them were heavy nursing cases, many of whom died shortly after admission. This was a great strain on the nursing staff. One female patient required four nurses to do her dressings and lift her in bed; many of her dressings had to be done under anaesthesia.

At first, only one wing had been opened, with three 4-bedded wards and three single rooms. As a routine was established, and the nursing staff began to acquire their own experience of nursing these special patients, so the second ward could be opened. Practical points were learnt – dessert spoons with rounded ends were replaced with pointed in order to aid feeding. Little idiosyncracies were tolerated – the large gentleman who insisted in storing his urine bottle in his equally large boots under his bed was allowed to continue this unconventional practice.

Gradually, thanks to earlier notification of need, the length of stay rose to an average of three weeks. All of them were of an urgent nature, although the number who were able to return home, albeit temporarily, continued to surprise and delight the nursing staff. Of the 275 patients admitted in the first year, 51 were discharged home for longer or shorter periods during their treatment. One of the chief benefits of St Barnabas' immediately became obvious – the giving of attentive, qualified care in the most appropriate surroundings. Dr. Gusterson was able to quote in his second newsletter the case of a patient who arrived very ill indeed

> but after a few days we were able to relieve the pain and find a suitable diet. Before long the patient was up for long periods of the day and eating almost a normal diet. She had many outside interests and one day she asked if she could have a committee meeting in her room! Two days later she was taken by car and chaired a meeting of that particular society!

He told that story 'pour encourager les autres' and part of his activity in the first years was to remind everyone of the potential for every patient to receive expert care, and knowing that some would indeed be able to return to their homes several times.

The care of patients was, of course, not restricted to medical and nursing attention. At a daily conference, Dr. Gusterson expressed his concern about the husband of a patient; he seemed unable to face the situation. However, a senior sister reported, 'He's all right now – I sat for half an hour with him on the edge of the fish-pond last night'. On another occasion, when Dr. Gusterson rang in about one male patient and asked how the others were faring, he was told, 'Oh, all the men are looking at the fight on television in the Day Room'. And Dr. Gusterson admitted one patient five months earlier than would have been normal because the fits which the patient was enduring might well have caused him to become threatening and violent towards his young family.

Sometimes the nursing staff described their work as a 'humbling experience' especially when relatives expressed their gratitude. One elderly lady held a coffee morning once a year in memory of her husband; another held an annual wine and cheese party, bringing in the money in a toffee tin, totalling more than £5,000 over the years.

The House Committee felt it necessary to appoint a deputy to Miss Sackse, the Matron. The first occupant of this post was Miss Margaret Stroud. Previously a staff nurse on a children's ward in the West Cornwall Hospital, she had heard about and studied the work of Dame Cecily Saunders at St Christopher's Hospice, and was ready to seize the opportunity to come to St Barnabas'. When Miss Sackse herself retired in March 1975 Miss Stroud automatically succeeded her and was herself succeeded by Sister D. Heptinstall.

On her retirement, Miss Sackse told the House Committee that the post had been the happiest and most rewarding of her professional career (she had received no salary at her own request). This was the tribute which the Council paid her:

> The whole conception of the work of St Barnabas' Home depends, not only upon medical and nursing skill of the highest order, but on a sensitive and spiritual conviction reaching beyond the immediate demands of nursing service. To this exacting requirement Miss Sackse has given herself with undeviating and selfless devotion. The atmosphere of quiet efficiency and serene and happy peacefulness, for which St Barnabas' is noted, is considerably due to the leadership and service of our first Matron, to whom we convey not only our profound thankfulness, but our warmest good wishes for her future.

In Chapter Two, brief mention was made of Dr. Jean Kay who acted as a locum from the time St Barnabas' opened. She had been a Houseman at the Royal Alexandra Hospital for Children in Brighton in 1972 when Dr. Gusterson visited as a locum anaesthetist. She heard about his plans for the Home and recalls:

> When Gus said he would be looking for two local GPs to help him run the new hospice, I told him I was starting as a GP in Arundel when I finished the Surgical House job in July 1972 ... Thus it was that on 18 January 1973 I started doing two half days a week at St Barnabas'. What Gus didn't then know was that I was pregnant – and as the bump got bigger the nurses called it 'little Barnabas'. On 17 April 1973 little Barnabas was born and six weeks later was the first babe to be baptised in the Home.

The baby was baptised by the Revd N. Evans, vicar of Durrington; the staff gave little Barnabas a replica of an antique spoon as a christening gift.

Dr. Kay's appointment relieved Dr. Gusterson of some of the burden of routine medical work and enabled him to be free one evening a week to see relatives of patients. The financial implication of her appointment would be to raise the bed cost by £1 per week (which sounds a very positive return on the investment!). The Home was already benefiting from locum support provided by the five doctors of the Heene Road Medical Practice, who gave three 3½-hour sessions per week plus cover on Tuesday nights, Friday (day and night) and alternate weekends. Dr. Gusterson was very happy with this arrangement because it had the real benefit of getting local practitioners involved in the work of the Home and he saw this as a vital step in its development.

One of the battles which took up much of Dr. Gusterson's time was that of making sure that local general practitioners knew exactly what the Home had to offer. He published the following statistics to illustrate his point:

	1973	1974	1975
Discharged to own home	51	21	41
Transferred to other N.H.	10	9	16
Died at St Barnabas'	214	208	226
Length of stay of patients (days):			
1-4	63	50	71
5-8	25	35	47
9-12	23	16	37
13-16	28	22	36
17-20	22	18	18
21-24	17	10	9
25-28	16	13	7
29-32	12	8	9
over 32 days, up to 100 days	67	56	42

Fifty-one patients had two stays, eight had three and one had four. His comment on the short stay of so many was that those patients were unable to benefit from the full resources available, namely pain relief and nursing care.

In February 1976, he reported to the House Committee that:

> he was still desperately worried about the complete lack of understanding of what this work was about, particularly amongst the medical profession. Recently, several more doctors had asked us to take patients who were almost unconscious and he was now having to say that we did not build this Home to provide somewhere for doctors to off-load their moribund patients.

Strong words, but we must remember that he was doing pioneering work in this field. So when a large local medical practice asked if their trainee assistant could spend a day at the Home, he was delighted to agree – this was one method of ensuring that they could 'get their work across' to the medical profession.

He had to rule, however, that some cases could not be admitted, for nursing rather than for compassionate reasons. He claimed that at least once a month he received a request from a social worker asking if the Home could take someone suffering from

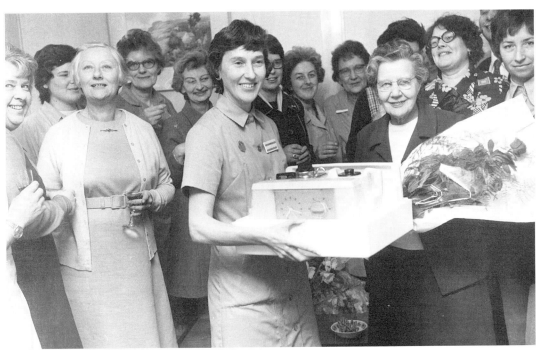

8   *Presentation by Miss Stroud to Miss Sackse on her retirement. (Photo:* Worthing Herald*)*

motor neurone disease, but they could not admit them owing to their very different nursing and care needs. (This policy was changed in January 1993.) Similarly, the question was raised whether they could admit cases of carcinoma when the patient was also senile and needed custodial care. Despite great pressure in one instance, they had refused on the grounds that it would interfere with 'our main work of rehabilitating patients and would have disturbed our other patients'. Nor could they take cases from the East Sussex Area Health Authority owing to the lack of any funding arrangement.

Visitors have always been welcome at St Barnabas' whatever the occasion. A newly-married couple once came to share tea with their aunt, a patient, before changing to leave for their honeymoon. One Christmas, a five-year-old ballet dancer came in to cheer Granny. The staff discovered the very real value of allowing family pets into the building. Dr. Gusterson described in his January 1977 newsletter how Robbie, a little dog, called every day to see his mistress. He would hop on to the bed and even, with the doctor turning a blind eye, snuggle down inside the sheets. The point was that this little dog was a great comfort to the patient. A 16-year-old patient had two guinea pigs brought in two or three times a week to romp on an 'inco' pad on her bed. Basically, this was all part of the process of making a patient feel at home.

One visitor who was always welcome at St Barnabas' was Lavinia, Duchess of Norfolk, who had become President following the death of Duke Bernard in 1975. She preferred many of her visits, usually at Easter, bringing Easter eggs for the patients, and Christmas, when she brought presents for the staff, to be as informal as possible. She enjoyed talking to the patients and the staff who found her so approachable and always to have a word of encouragement. Whenever possible, she would be

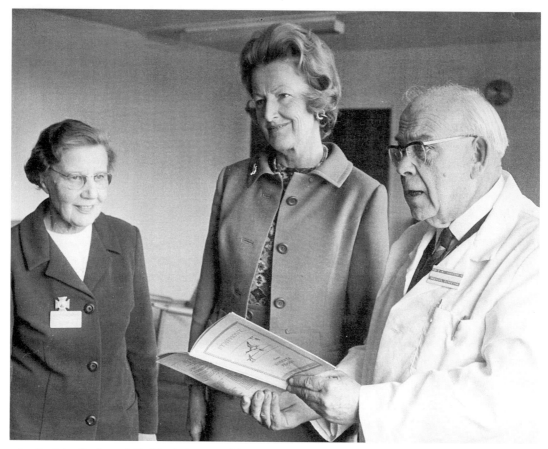

9 *Lavinia, Duchess of Norfolk during one of her many visits, with Miss Sackse, Matron and Dr. Gusterson.*

accompanied by her dogs, which themselves gave great pleasure to the patients. (After her death in 1995, she was succeeded by her daughter, Lady Sarah Clutton, who has continued the tradition of visiting. Her golden retriever, however, on one visit caused some alarm by deciding to take a dip in the fish-pond!)

The question of payment of fees was one of the thorniest issues which had to be faced. We have seen how Dr. Gusterson had assured everyone that any patient who needed care would not be excluded on grounds of inability to pay. This promise was always kept but establishing the ability to pay at such a traumatic time in the life of the patient and family was a delicate process. One solution was to suggest that any contribution made by patients should be assessed in two parts – first, any contribution to the weekly bed costs, even if that were only, say, £15-20 per week and secondly, to suggest that some settlement of the total cost could be made from the patient's estate. This was acceptable to most families. The significant role played by legacies in the income of St Barnabas' over its 25 years is perhaps rooted in this compassionate concept. (Owing to all these difficulties, the question of the payment of fees was dropped in 1975.)

In the realm of finance, the trustees were exploring uncharted territory. As they gradually discovered at first hand the problems associated with running a Home of this size and nature, alternating cries of relief and panic echo through the Minutes of the House Committee and the Council (at this time). In July 1974 one such minute records that 'running St Barnabas' Home was now "big business"' and those overseeing the finances admitted that they were working from day to day. Three monthly items were giving particular concern: wages (£4,800), laundry (£280), National Health and Graduated Pensions (£320), totalling £5,400 for these three items alone, led them to describe their outgoings as 'tremendous' (we must recall that in 1998 values this was about £45,000 per month). The most significant item of revenue, which could at least be planned for, was the payment by the Hospital Board for the contracted beds based on a bed cost of £7.30 per day, but the payments were made in arrears and over £6,700 was overdue. Also at this time, £3,000 was owing from the NSCR and £3,500 from the estates of deceased patients. To compound the issue, it was discovered that a threshold increase on the Whitley scale should have been paid to all staff (except the doctors and administration staff). A new pay circular, received in the following December, meant that about £20 per bed per week was added to the costs. By the end of 1974, the monthly outgoings were in the order of £8,500 putting the annual turnover at over £100,000. For about seven months that year, the income was £700-£800 short of the amount needed to meet running costs. (Curiously, a note in the Minute Book of the House Committee records that the Bursar had gone on holiday; the funds were sufficient 'to pay for just two weeks' wages, and nothing else, and the cheque book had been hidden'!)

As the Home began its new accounting year (1975), one of the most encouraging aspects was the amount received in donations in the previous financial year. These were sources over which the Committee had no control. Donations in lieu of flowers from St Barnabas' patients were £6,470 and from others £2,767; pure and special donations and responses to newsletters totalled £15,300. These three items themselves were sufficient to support nearly five beds for one year.

We have seen how, at a very early stage, Dr. Gusterson and Dr. Franks had established contact with the local and area Health Authorities. The most significant, tangible benefit was to agree Authority funding for a specified number of contractual beds. The beneficiaries were not only St Barnabas' with a guaranteed source of income but also the Authority, who were able to direct patients to St Barnabas' who might otherwise have been occupying hospital beds. This contractual arrrangement was perhaps the most important of the financial securities which enabled the Home to remain financially viable.

In the Spring of the following year, Mr. Bradwell, the Bursar, reported that he had been in touch with the new Area Health Authority about the desirability of increasing the amount paid for each contractual bed. Sadly, he was unable to conclude his negotiations, as he died suddenly in September. His successor, Mr. Edwin Berry, was able to take the negotiations further with the result that from 1 November 1975 the payment made by the Authority was increased from £105 to £115.50 per week. Mr. Berry also introduced a more sophisticated system of tracking bed costs based on a daily cost figure which enabled adjustments to be made as costs fluctuated.

In March 1977 the Council discussed the question of additional medical assistance. A small sub-committee was set up to investigate and recommended the appointment of a physician. This was offered to Dr. Alan Kingsbury from the Heene Road practice, to be effective from 1 October 1977. Dr. Gusterson told the Council that, as physician, his work would cover the medical side and that in time Dr. Kingsbury would come to know the administrative aspects, too. Asked whether Dr. Kingsbury should understudy Dr. Gusterson, the doctor replied that 'it would be impossible to differentiate in detail' and suggested 'that the situation should be left to grow, as it naturally will'.

In January 1977 Dr. George Deutsch, consultant in radiotherapy and oncology at the Royal Sussex County Hospital, who had been most helpful in advising about treatment to patients in St Barnabas', was formally appointed Honorary Consultant, thus bringing additional expertise to the Home. He was to remain actively involved with St Barnabas' until February 1998.

Some very welcome news came in a letter from the Area Health Authority following a half-yearly inspection:

> Registration of Nursing Homes – Nursing Homes Act 1975
>
> I write on behalf of the Area Health Authority following Mrs. Franklin's visit to St Barnabas' on 24 January, 1977. I have no need to tell you that you have a very well run home with high standards of patient care and that you do indeed provide an excellent service. It is however pleasant to record officially such a fact and also to note how friendly and efficient the staff are which gives a peaceful pleasant atmosphere throughout the home.
>
> One item from Mrs. Franklin's remarks, however, deserves special mention and that is your developing service to visit patients in the community to provide the link for urgent admission if and when this becomes necessary.

A perceptive comment which indicated one of the most important aspects of care which St Barnabas' was to develop.

The NSCR gave valuable support and encouragement to St Barnabas' from its formative stage. It supported financially five beds at £85 per week up to 1978. When, however, the Council discussed Dr. Gusterson's proposal to make a loan for a Home to be built in the Horsham/Crawley area, they realised that this would not have met with the approval of the NSCR. They also realised that their financial position, thanks mainly to legacies, was such that the NSCR might want to cease their support, and so they wrote to them accordingly. At the same time, Mr. Roe wrote to the local branch of the Society expressing thanks for the wonderful support which they had given from the inception of the appeal. In his newsletter of July 1978, Dr. Gusterson paid tribute to the Society:

> In the early years we were most grateful to the National Society for Cancer Relief who not only gave us a capital grant towards the building cost but also an annual grant. That Society is now heavily committed in helping to start other units and we therefore offered to forego our grant on the understanding that we can call on them if we cannot meet our expenses. This means that we shall have to find at least another £26,000 a year but we feel that our friends will stand by us.

In the meantime Dr. Gusterson was also working on a wider front. The demands on his time from outside the Home gradually increased and so there developed a distinct missionary element to his activities.

He was host to visitors from this country, from Europe and Scandinavia, the USA and the Antipodes. Those who came were usually wanting to start similar homes, in such diverse places as Bath, Bristol, Durham, Eastbourne, Falkirk, Horsham and Crawley, Lancaster, Lincoln, Milton Keynes, Newcastle-upon-Tyne and St Austell. They were interested in the standard of nursing care, the financing and the design of the building.

He found this stimulating, and hard work: 'our problem was trying to create the correct image of the type of work we did here and these visits enabled us to share our ideas. The best description which evolved was "teaching people to learn to live with malignancy"'.

Overseas visitors came from the USA, Japan, Holland, Sweden, New Zealand and Germany. The greatest number were from the USA where, at that time, there was only one residential hospice in the whole country. Fund-raisers, doctors, medical historians, nurses, priests, researchers and social workers were among the visitors. The Americans were particularly struck by the calm atmosphere of St Barnabas', the construction of the building and, repeatedly, the bed pan disposal unit which was not available in the USA. Those from Germany described how difficult it would be to integrate such care into the German Health Service where there was serious resistance to change in medical thinking on terminal care; the churches, much more heavily involved in social work, were more likely to take the initiative. Yet a visitor from Hong Kong surprised him by saying that they had a 180-bed hospital devoted to the care of advanced cases of cancer. A party of nurses from Stockholm left the nursing staff the gift of a Tea Light; and 35 German geriatric nurses showed their appreciation by making a collection and presenting a cheque for £127.

Dr. Gusterson was also a regular speaker at conferences. One such was run by the Religious Society of Friends (Quakers) at Dorking on terminal care; in Dortmund, Germany, he spoke on the same subject and in Guernsey on pain management, finding the experience 'high-powered but worthwhile'. He addressed a group of 30 hospital chaplains in Sheffield describing it as 'a profitable time'. He opened a series of lectures at Kent University on 'Current Attitudes to Death and Bereavement' and spoke at a conference run by The Royal Society of Health on 'The Need of the National Health Service for Private Nursing Homes' (would Mr. Gisby have approved?). He was always honoured to be invited to conferences sponsored by St Christopher's Hospice where he made many of his international contacts. (Dr. Gusterson's energy was necessarily often expended on the road; in December 1979 he was fined £6 by Worthing magistrates for speeding at 41mph in Offington Lane. He pleaded that he was following a van in the line of traffic ahead, and assumed they were all within the law!)

One invitation he received gave him great delight – it was to one of the Queen's Garden Parties at Buckingham Palace in July 1976. Afterwards, he described the experience as being 'quite out of this world and one which provided a glimpse of quiet, gracious and dignified living'. One wonders whether he realised that his work was directed to exactly the same ends for those who came to St Barnabas'.

He was not afraid of taking on controversial subjects, as when he took part in a public discussion in Hove with the Chairman of the Exit Group on the subject of euthanasia on which he had strong views. When Malcolm Muggeridge and Alan Thornhill wrote a play 'Sentenced to Life' as a challenge to those who advocated 'mercy killing', he produced a leaflet giving information in terminal care.

He took the opportunity to speak about the Home on 'Thought for the Day' on Radio Brighton. His published text shows so clearly his love and compassion as well as his Christian conviction. (He produced a little book of prayers for use at St Barnabas' by patients and friends, which must have brought consolation to many people.)

All this national and international activity did not stop him from keeping his feet very much on the ground. This was evidenced by the questions and points of detail which he could raise at committee meetings. What was being done about the excessive number of daisies in the grass? Why was it necessary to buy new wallpaper for the Day Room when he understood that the paper was washable? He was worried about the packet of dried yeast and the equipment which had disappeared from the flower bay – could not a simple partition be put up to make the area less accessible? He was concerned about the constant parking of 'enormous lorries' by the entrance to St Barnabas' and by the excessive amounts of rainwater which tended to accumulate in the visitors' car park. On another occasion he was concerning himself with the ventilating hood and extractor fan in the kitchen, as the temperature had reached 90°, and how to replace the tired old musical box which used to play 'Happy Birthday' over the tannoy whenever a patient had a birthday. (He might have cast his mind back to May 1974 when he showed anxiety about the lack of any fire drill procedures in spite of representations to the Fire Brigade. By September, a procedure had been agreed, but not before the Brigade had had to respond to an alarm when a sensor activated the alarm bells. They arrived in just under four minutes to discover that the sensor had been set off by an earwig! And during one drill a voice was heard from behind a curtained bed: 'What am I supposed to do? I'm on the commode'.)

One of the most poignant minutes of the Council is that of 18 September 1979 referring to the recent death of Mrs. Gusterson:

> The Council ... desires to record its thankfulness for the life of Mrs. Dorothy Gusterson. She died, as she had lived, graciously, peacefully and radiating a calm assurance, offering selfless service, which helped all who knew her and which, in the tremendous days of the founding of St Barnabas' Home was of the utmost assistance and inspiration, particularly to her husband, our Medical Director. While aware of his steadfast Christian faith and courage at this time, the Council conveys to him and his family its profound sympathy in their personal loss.

The Council then stood in silent memory. In thanking them for their tribute, Dr. Gusterson said that it was largely due to his wife that he had accepted the challenge to become Chairman of the original steering committee. As his daughter, Jane, later commented: 'The fact that Dorothy could come into St Barnabas' during her illness made it all worthwhile for my father'.

Mrs. Gusterson had touched the lives of many people. One very tangible way was in the evergreen arrangements in St Barnabas' which were her speciality for the winter months, and staff still recall how she supported her husband in the physical preparations of the Home even to the cost of their own Christmas celebrations.

It was around this time that some members of the Council were expressing concern about the number of hours Dr. Gusterson was putting in at the Home. His pastoral care meant that he would seldom miss an evening visit to each patient after his day's work, visits that were valued by the patients. But his colleagues could see the effect on his health and, after his return from hospital following his first heart attack, they urged him to 'take things more easily'. It has to be said that, in spite of his active life, he still found time for his hobbies which included photography and gardening, an interest which he had shared very much with his wife. The 700 alpine plants in his garden, which he used to open to the public from time to time, were each meticulously tagged, and holidays walking in the Swiss mountains provided an opportunity to discover new varieties. He also collected antique pewter.

Inevitably, the question of his retirement had to arise. The Council met on 6 January 1981 to ask for his comments. His response was recorded thus:

> He understood that the Sub-committee saw a need for fundamental changes in the administration of the Home and he had every confidence in handing over the medical work to Dr. Kingsbury. He said that he would be 75 in a few days' time and suggested that the 31st January would be an appropriate time for him to retire. He went on to say that he would always be willing to do what he could in the best interests of St Barnabas'. This was then discussed and his resignation accepted 'with deep understanding'. He was immediately elected as Vice-President with a seat on the Council.

It is fair to say that he made his resignation with reluctance; it is not difficult to appreciate that his involvement with St Barnabas' had been so deep that to break his attachment was a painful experience for him.

A sherry party was held on 30 January to mark his retirement. He was presented with two books, *English Abbeys and Cathedrals* and a book by the illustrator of *Winnie the Pooh*, and a selection of choice wines.

When the Council met on 24 February, one of the items on its agenda was the question of a testimonial to Dr. Gusterson, who was present. When his views were invited, he replied that the tribute paid to him by his successor, Dr. Kingsbury, was sufficient. But the Chairman, Mr. Roe, said that he could not leave without a show of appreciation. A suggestion had been made by the physiotherapist, Miss Nash, that a pastel of Dr. Gusterson, to be hung in the Home, should be commissioned from the artist Juliet Pannett. On 30 April, at a small reception at the Home, the President, Her Grace Lavinia, Duchess of Norfolk, presented him with the pastel portrait, and a 17th-century William and Mary pewter tankard. 'Gus' graciously agreed that the portrait could hang in the entrance hall of the Home, where it can still be seen today.

His work for the hospice movement nationally and internationally, as well as at St Barnabas', led him to be awarded the Cross of Honour of the Sovereign Order of St John of Jerusalem. This was presented to him at the Annual Investiture Service of the Order in St Botolph's Without Bishopgate, London on 4 April 1981.

Just five months later, on 11 September 1981, Dr. Gusterson died peacefully in his sleep.

Dr. Kingsbury, who had come to know him so well and to value so highly the experience of working closely with 'Gus', paid this tribute to him in the next newsletter:

> He was a man of remarkable vision who saw the need for establishing a Home like St Barnabas' and a man of even more remarkable determination and fortitude to bring about the realisation of that vision.
>
> He had a delightful sense of humour, occasionally at his own expense and often used to quote the following from W.H. Auden's 'Shorts':
>
> > Give me a doctor, partridge plump,
> > Short in the leg and broad in the rump,
> > An endomorph with gentle hands
> > Who'll never make absurd demands
> > That I abandon all my vices,
> > Nor pull a long face in a crisis
> > But with a twinkle in his eye
> > Will tell me that I have to die.
>
> Those of us who knew him well suspect that he would really like this as his epitaph. Above all, he was a spiritual man. Although a 'non-Conformist' in his faith, as in all that he was and did, he eventually found his place within the Anglican tradition and his commitment to the Church of England was total, being made a Diocesan Lay Reader in 1972. He was actively employed

10 Letter of condolence from the Duchess of Norfolk

in the work of the Church and Hospice movement to the end. He died peacefully in his sleep; the books at his bedside were the Bible and Hans Kung's 'On Being a Christian'.

Dr. Gusterson's funeral was held at Storrington Church on 18 September. His daughters, Jane and Elizabeth, received a personal letter from the Duchess of Norfolk who had come to know 'Gus' so well.

A Thanksgiving Service, on 6 November 1981 at St Paul's Church, Worthing, was attended by over 400 people, in the presence of his family, friends, close colleagues and staff of St Barnabas' Home and representatives from seven other hospices in England. The lessons were read by his son-in-law, Commander J. Harvey-Samuel RN and the Matron, Miss M.E. Stroud. A Personal Word was given by Dr. Kingsbury and the Address by Canon J.W. Reeves. The hymns included 'Who would true valour see' and 'God be in my head' which, sung kneeling, concluded the service. But perhaps the final word should come from Dr. Gusterson himself. In the newsletter in which he announced his retirement, he quoted as his farewell the prayer of Sir Francis Drake:

> O Lord God when thou givest to thy servants to endeavour any great matter, grant us also to know that it is not in the beginning, but the continuing of the same until it be thoroughly finished which yieldeth the true Glory.

That prayer is an eloquent tribute to his achievements.

CHAPTER 4

EXPANSION

The transition to the new leadership of Dr. Kingsbury was achieved smoothly, not least because he had been so close to Dr. Gusterson for over three years. He was known and respected by the staff, and in spite of claiming that 'it was a somewhat daunting prospect to step into Dr. Gusterson's shoes', a man 'vibrant, enthusiastic and full of vigour' he soon demonstrated that he had his own inspiration and vision for the future of St Barnabas'. With the firm foundations put in place by Dr. Gusterson, he was ideally placed to develop the potential for growth and to build on the strengths of the Home, not least its reputation for care and compassion. As one patient put it:

> You are all so kind and attentive, you make us feel just like one of the family, no matter what you do for us, or ask us to do for ourselves, we are confident and secure knowing it is for our own good.

In-patient care, the purpose for which the Home was designed and built, was, of course, the most important part of the work. But the staffing levels were sometimes under pressure, as in September 1982 when, with 27 patients in the Home, and with some of them requiring a lot of specialised care, Sister Heptinstall commented that 'the staff have been working to their limit physically and emotionally with the holiday season in full swing'. Two members of the nursing staff were on maternity leave, another had resigned for family reasons. The laundry lady had been off sick for seven weeks and this had placed extra work on the nursing staff. The relief kitchen cook had also been sick for two weeks. During one week, they were unable to have any admissions for these reasons. To make matters even worse, the washing machines were giving trouble, one being out of action for three weeks while another was leaking very badly. The Matron had to advertise for trained and auxiliary staff. Occasionally, staff suffered verbal or physical abuse from a patient. A staff nurse was punched in the eye and was off sick for ten days. The staff realised that patients sometimes 'do not know what they are doing' but such incidents were always reported to the House Committee. On another occasion, no admissions were possible for six days because there was a shortage of the equivalent of four full-time nurses due to sickness and family reasons, courses and holidays. However, after the sixth day, 16 patients were admitted in 10 days. It sometimes happened, too, that one of their own number died in their care, as when Miss Rosemary Cummings died after seven years' service as a nursing auxiliary and staff nurse J. Hazelden after several years service to St Barnabas'. (The dedication of the staff emerges in a quaint request by Miss Stroud one February, that 'something might be done to combat the effects of ice on the drive, as several staff had fallen off their bicycles recently through skidding on black ice early in the morning'.) Additionally, as the building programme developed and extensions of varying sizes were added or alterations made, the staff had to cope with workmen on site, with up to five different firms at the same time. (Sometimes this had its humorous side. Returning from lunch one day during a redecoration project, a Sister heard heavy snoring in one of the empty ward bays. Opening the door, she saw a workman, still wearing his heavy boots, sound asleep on the bed enjoying a post-prandial siesta!) And in the earlier days when the flat roof leaked at the slightest opportunity, nurses had to dodge the buckets which were catching the dripping rain, having entered the roof space many feet away from its exit point.

Yet the work of caring continued and Dr. Kingsbury instigated a series of staff discussions, trying to create an openness and giving time and opportunity to review questions and concerns.

From these discussions, some interesting points arose from the staff who said that they would like:

1. A greater knowledge and understanding of the Funding of the Home
2. A greater understanding of modern treatments available
3. A greater understanding of bereavement
4. More information, if possible, about patients who have been discharged from the Home; possibly in the form of a daily bulletin to be posted in the staff room
5. Badges for staff; the St Barnabas' logo could be used to create a badge about the size of a 1 or 2 pence piece
6. A piano for the pleasure of patients and staff alike.

With the statutory requirement for the registration of nursing homes taking patients with a terminal illness, came the need to conform to the staffing levels which this legislation set out.

One result was that there had to be two trained nurses on duty at all times, thus requiring the hiring of four additional staff even though this would not raise any additional income. It is also instructive to note from the minutes of the House Committee and the Council that salary awards were always honoured (even if they may not have been budgeted), a sure sign of the confidence in and appreciation of the staff.

In January 1988 the House Committee had a lengthy discussion to see how the problems about recruitment might be overcome, perhaps by improving facilities for nurses, by enabling part-time employees to benefit from a pension scheme (which might cost around £15,000 a year) or by payment for unsocial hours. At one stage the House Committee considered purchasing a house adjacent to St Barnabas' to offer accommodation with a view to attracting staff. The idea was dropped when it was discovered that a restrictive covenant on the local estate would not permit such a use of a property.

On the question of pensions, anomalies sometimes arose when staff who had transferred from the NHS were able to bring their pension rights with them, and these were often more favourable than the scheme in existence. After careful investigation, it was ruled that the Home would adopt the scheme known as the Federated Pension Scheme, and employees could opt for the scheme which was most beneficial to them.

The lady who had led the nursing team through these years of change, Miss Margaret Stroud, retired in 1988 after 13 years' service. Dr. Kingsbury paid her this tribute:

EXPANSION

The quantity and quality of service that she has given to the Hospice is acknowledged by all who knew her. Over the years there have probably been many members of staff who would not have been able to continue work in the Hospice at some time or other without Matron's encouragement and support. I number myself as one of them and I have counted it an enormous privilege to have had the opportunity of working with her and to know her friendship.

Her successor was Miss M. 'Bobby' Chapman. Unfortunately, she was taken seriously ill in the following May and only returned home from hospital in July. She died after taking early retirement. Miss Heather Fittock, the Clinical Teacher, who had been deputising for her during her absence, was appointed Matron in November 1989.

To return now to Dr. Kingsbury's vision for the Home. These are the priorities he described to the House Committee:

1 Education – The means of getting the message across to the Community and to hospitals of the work that is done here, particularly to nurses and doctors
2 Home Care – The visiting of patients who go home from here, and also the visiting of the bereaved
3 Volunteers who are prepared to assist where necessary
4 Day Centre – The possibility of this being available in the Home, which would also be of benefit to the In-Patients.

In 1978 both he and Dr. Gusterson had advocated strongly to the House Committee for the provision of a conference room, describing it as 'a necessity because we were being asked to do more and more explaining of our work to people in the

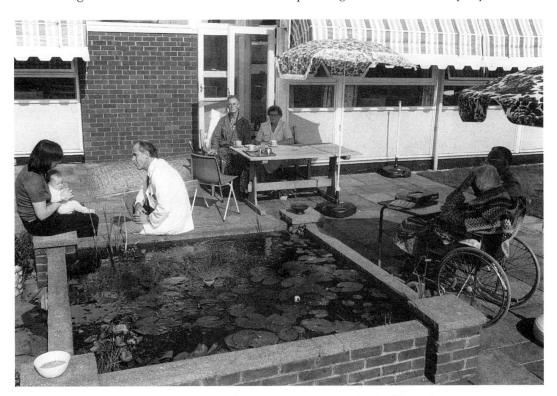

11   *Dr. Kingsbury talks to a very young visitor by the fish-pond*

medical, nursing and social fields'. Some members were concerned about the impact of visitors on the quiet atmosphere of the Home but, with others feeling that the Home should be sharing its knowledge and expertise, their counsel prevailed.

Dr. Kingsbury's enthusiasm for education was evident and his ideas received a thorough and lengthy analysis by the House Committee and the Council. The decision fully to support him was given and was never to waver.

The main plank of his proposals concerned his wish to provide training both for the staff of the Home and also of other units, the latter with the objective of furthering the understanding of the care of patients with a terminal illness.

The staff of the In Service and Post Basic Training department of the Worthing and Southlands School of Nursing had prepared an outline syllabus on 'Care of the Dying' for the Joint Board Clinical Studies Nursing Course, and it was hoped that members of the staff would eventually attend the six-week course so that they would all hold the JBCNS certificate. To ensure that their training would be achieved and be of an acceptable standard, Dr. Kingsbury sought the agreement of the Council to appoint a clinical teacher who would be responsible for the in-service training of staff. The Council agreed, having heard that the NSCR had agreed to finance the appointment for three years. The cost of advertising the post was met by the Worthing Group of Hospitals and it was subsequently awarded to Mr. Trevor Caddick, who joined the staff as Macmillan Clinical Teacher on 3 January 1983. In May, Mr. Caddick attended a meeting of the House Committee to describe the outline of the first course to be held in June for a period of six weeks. Lecturers had been arranged to speak on various topics and members of trained staff in the Home would be welcome to take part in the lectures if workload permitted. He agreed that it would be uppermost in everyone's mind that the care of the patients came first and that the students, who would be clearly badged, would always be working with trained members of staff.

The real feather in Mr. Caddick's cap came with the running of a course in the 'Care of the Dying Patient' under the auspices of the English National Board, whose aims were to provide in-service training for nurses in a wide range of disciplines. The first course turned out to be a success. It was attended by five trained nurses, including one of the Sisters from St Barnabas'. The measure of its success was partly evident on the last day when each student presented a project on which they had been working. Dr. Kingsbury declared these to be of a very high standard, and Miss Stroud complimented Mr. Caddick on the planning of the course and his contribution to its success. Thus was established an aspect of St Barnabas' which was to play an increasingly important part in its care programme.

The next course was also a success. Attended by six post-graduate nurses from Chichester, Shoreham and Worthing, including not only community nurses but a Night Sister, a Ward Sister and a Stoma Care nurse, the Matron was again enthusiastic. By the beginning of 1985 the course was well established and, importantly, fully accepted by the nursing staff who were glad to welcome the nurses to St Barnabas'. (Later, similar provision was made for a course in the 'Care of the Elderly', also under the auspices of the ENB.)

These successes had a sad ending. Trevor Caddick died suddenly at the age of 36 on 18 March 1985 whilst on holiday with his parents. In his time at St Barnabas' he had not only set up training programmes but had been actively engaged in the home care work. Dr. Kingsbury spoke warmly of his work, which had been seminal:

> He had been concerned with all student visits, mainly pupil nurses in training at local hospitals, and also with other visitors to the Home. He had been involved in the education of St Barnabas' staff and had organised lectures. He played a major role in the English National Board course held twice yearly for six weeks. On the Home Care side he had been responsible for all patients who had returned home and these could number from 40 to 70. He had also been responsible for bereavement visits and this involved between 200/250 visits a year. When necessary, he had also made pre-admission visits.

When Dr. Kingsbury asked the Council for their approval to appoint a replacement clinical teacher who would also be responsible for the day care unit and home care visiting, they unanimously agreed. This was a fitting memorial to Mr. Caddick's work.

In July, Miss Heather Fittock, who was the clinical teacher at Southlands, began her work as his successor. The courses continued to be successful, with nurses from differing backgrounds attending. They gained an overall view of hospice care, they read and studied away from their working environment and could return to their units able to spread ideas to help patients with a terminal illness. As the courses developed, so Miss Fittock was able to draw on assistance from additional tutors. The education effort was expanded to include study days for general practitioners, district nurses and hospital nurses. Many of these students were to come from overseas. The CRUSE organisation later began to use the facilities for their courses.

Dr. Kingsbury's second objective concerned home care. (The first record of this area of work being mentioned in any Minutes is as far back as March 1974, when Dr. Gusterson was looking forward to Sister M. Gray joining the staff in August. She was a former Deputy Matron and then Matron at the Zachary Merton Hospital (succeeding Miss C. Grose who had, on retirement, joined St Barnabas' as a ward Sister). She would be engaged on following up patients who had gone home and keeping in touch with relatives, especially the alone husband or wife. These visits proved to be successful, and she gave some excellent reports on the patients. So successful was she, that in 1976 she visited 276 patients at home and 82 bereaved relatives. Her circuit had ranged from Bognor Regis to West Chiltington and Shoreham-by-Sea and she had travelled 759 miles. In the following year, the House Committee was ready to agree that a further increase in staffing was necessary to ensure that this service was adequately maintained.)

When Dr. Kingsbury presented his ideas for home care, he wrote:

> It has become increasingly evident that this role is not to provide direct nursing for the patient but support for those who are providing the direct care. That is advice and encouragement to the General Practitioners, Community Nurses, Social Services personnel and above all, to the relatives and/or friends who provide all that is necessary for the patient twenty-four hours a day, seven days a week. We should not, and indeed cannot, take on these vital roles which they can play but we can, when we are called upon, assist and advise them with our expertise in symptom control and nursing procedures.

Local meetings with these professional carers had been fruitful. Mr. Caddick, with Sister E. Lawson, Sister H. Morley and Sister Gray, had 39 patients who were being regularly visited; they also aimed to make at least one visit to the bereaved. The particular value of this proposed service was that those from St Barnabas' had the knowledge, the information and the time – the focused care – which for a busy GP or district nurse was often impossible. (The relationship between Home Care nurses and district nurses was an important one, and gradually strengthened as mutual trust and respect were built up.)

In July 1984 Dr. Kingsbury put to the Council a case for the appointment of a full-time sister to work in the Home Care team. He wanted to broaden the work in the community especially supporting people remaining in their own homes, of which there could be 40 to 60 at any one time.

In July 1987 he and Dr. Ruddle were confident that the service should be expanded to all patients who came on to the Home's books and that the Home Care team should be developed and increased in size. (It was to grow to eight by 1998.) They told the Council that the Team was continuing to provide a counselling and advisory service to patients in their own homes on referral by him, but a direct nurse to nurse referral of patients was being set up. This was particularly for patients who would never need in-patient or day care by the St Barnabas' unit, and in the last six months there had been 15 such referrals.

In January 1988 Dr. Kingsbury was sure that this was a service which was bound to expand. When the service had begun, the number of pre-admission patients was 34 but this had now increased to 88. This was far too high a figure for two Sisters to visit effectively. The regularity of visits depended on the needs of individual patients and their families, some being visited daily, others weekly or once a month. The Chairman of Council, Mr. East, pointed out that in effect the Home would be providing additional resources for the district nursing service, but they were unlikely to gain any financial support from the local Health Authority. By 1989, the team consisted of four Sisters, and one third of the deaths recorded at St Barnabas' had occurred in patients' own homes. Two years later, the number of Sisters was six. Dr. Kingsbury felt that one of the consequences of this support was that the idea of the Hospice was now more acceptable to younger patients with young families.

(At this point, the change of name should be noted. In April 1987 the House Committee had discussed the possibility of changing the name to St Barnabas' Hospice, deleting 'Nursing Home' from the title. This was because the work of the hospice movement was now more widely known, and the change might well 'attract the financial sympathies of those persons who wish to assist financially with our aims'. It was felt that the title should convey the real task of St Barnabas', which might not be clear using the title 'Nursing Home'. The title 'Hospice' was generally used from this time although the formal change was only agreed at the Annual General Meeting on 28 November 1995.)

Dr. Kingsbury was eager to encourage the work of volunteers as his third priority. Dr. Gusterson had been lukewarm about their value but had instigated the provision of a trolley shop, having seen the effectiveness of the ladies who organised the flower rota. The trolley shop had been taken under the wing of Mrs. Nancy Lephard, a member of the House Committee, and she had turned it into a popular and successful enterprise.

EXPANSION

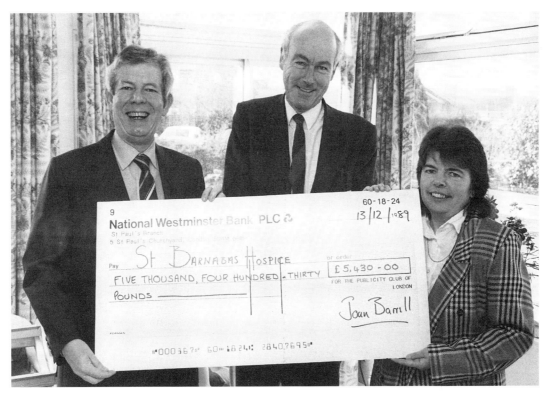

12 *Derek Jameson presents a cheque in appreciation of the care shown for his mother, who died at St Barnabas'. Francis de Beer, Bursar and Val Wells, Home Care Sister are smiling recipients.*

A gradual swell of interest developed, from people who had experienced the compassion shown to their relatives or who just wished to be of service in the community. It was some time before this goodwill was effectively harnessed, but that became the task of Mrs. Patricia Bowles, appointed Co-ordinator of Volunteers in 1983. At that time they numbered about seventy, and included the ladies who arranged the flowers, organised the tea trolley, together with the library service and the shop, all on a rota basis. The next development was for a daily rota for transport to bring patients to the Home when they had no transport of their own or where public transport was unavailable; it was not long before every day of the month was covered, with one or two drivers on standby for emergencies.

There was a need for volunteers to be in the Home on weekday mornings for what were described as 'General Duties' – helping in the kitchen with the patients' drinks, providing coffee for visiting relatives and also befriending them. Opportunities also existed for helping in the evenings in support of the supper cook and the nursing staff, and similarly at weekends. It was also envisaged that the volunteers could play a part in fund-raising. With Mrs. Joan Hunter working alongside her, Mrs. Bowles encouraged and developed this aspect of St Barnabas'.

An appeal for volunteers was made in the autumn of 1985, and 40 new volunteers were quickly integrated into the work of the Home. Their main value was in helping to support the running of the Day Centre; more drivers were recruited to cope with the extra demand for transport. Without the volunteers, the Centre would have been extremely restricted in its ability to care. The most difficult rota to fill was that for the kitchen in the evening; 'ladies without their own transport do not like to come out on dark evenings'. Some volunteers were not suitable for work in the Home, but were very keen to be considered for working in a charity shop if ever that were set up.

Mrs. Bowles and Mrs. Hunter were by now spending a great deal of time in the Home co-ordinating these activities. The latter once had the opportunity to show some Australian visitors around the Home; they were thinking of setting up their own volunteer system in Western Australia. The Minutes of the House Committee are liberally sprinkled with expressions of gratitude to these two ladies for their energy and work, and it is not surprising that, by the end of 1986, the House Committee had decided to appoint a full-time organiser. Mrs. Lysbeth Macrae took up her duties at the end of March 1987, reporting to Mr. Francis de Beer, the Administrator. By this time there were nearly 200 volunteers on board. With the numbers being so satisfactory, some volunteers were able to take patients down to the sea and have a morning coffee, as well as to help in the Day Centre.

Some volunteers would be directed towards activities where their own particular experience or skills could be used. Two such were Mr. Ken Hammond and Mrs. Anne Cox who were asked to help with bereavement visiting under the guidance of Sue Ramsey, the Home Care Sister with special bereavement responsibility. Within two months, they were each making two or three visits a week, learning to listen and to befriend as visitors, not counsellors. Through the stories they heard – ranging from tragic to comic – and the courage they saw, they both found the experience enriching. Their ability to help the bereaved to adjust to a traumatic change in their lives was a splendid example of the care which St Barnabas' felt it was its mission to offer, and this was often crowned when the bereaved came back for afternoon tea or another social occasion. This support was to be enhanced under the experienced eye of Julia Franklin who, with her experience in family situations and her extensive knowledge of the benefits structure, was appointed as the first Social Worker in 1989.

A fourth priority area of Dr. Kingsbury was that of the Day Centre concept. The original idea of the Home was, of course, that patients would enter for treatment and care for as long as they needed it; there was an underlying assumption that they were regarded as 'in-patients'. However, at a meeting of the House Committee as early as July 1976 Mrs. Bowles had asked about the possibility of opening a Day Centre, as this might well help to allay the reluctance of some people to come into St Barnabas'.

Dr. Kingsbury's experiences in working alongside Dr. Gusterson and in being encouraged by Mrs. Bowles had led him to conclude that at a Day Centre the quality of a patient's palliative care and symptom control could be monitored without the necessity for in-patient admission. Also it would introduce the patient to the Hospice and its staff in a relaxed and informal environment, whilst giving their carers at home a well-earned few hours' rest. Steps were taken to enlarge the Day Room and provide new offices and a bathroom so that full day-care facilities could be provided. In February 1985 a special meeting of the Council looked at the idea in some detail, including the proposals from the building consultant, Mr. J.C. Barrass. Dr. Kingsbury gave the Council members the opportunity to discuss all aspects, including staffing, costs and the impact of the building work. Their unanimous decision was to go ahead at a cost 'within 10 per cent of £70,000'. This would be met out of resources, and the new room would be called the 'day care unit'. The contract was awarded to J.C. Snelling, a well known Chichester firm.

While the building work was in progress one ward had to be closed, thus slightly reducing the number of admissions. By December, Dr. Kingsbury could report that the Day Centre was proving very popular both with in-patients and out-patients. Experience of running the Centre, however, showed that there was a need for someone to be appointed to 'act as Co-ordinator between all parties involved' in its running. It was thought that the appointment of an occupational therapist would be appropriate but that proved to be unworkable. The result was that much of the workload fell on Mrs. Tricia Bowles and Mrs. Joan Hunter. Eventually, it was thought that a professional nurse might be better suited to that work, someone who could liaise well with patients, drivers and volunteers. A staff nurse, Mrs. Jennifer Taylor, was subsequently appointed. From November 1985 up to ten patients attended on three days a week with plans to increase that to five days. The Centre was much appreciated and the volunteers had been a great asset especially with the expanding need for transport. By October 1986 the Centre was open for four days a week and proving to be great success.

But the highlight for patients and staff alike occurred on Friday, 29 November 1985 when the Centre was officially opened by Her Royal Highness, Diana Princess of Wales. The helicopter of the Queen's Flight landed in Palatine Park where Her Royal Highness was greeted by Lavinia, Duchess of Norfolk and Lord Lieutenant of West Sussex and President of St Barnabas' Home, together with the High Sheriff, Major-General Sir Philip Ward, the Mayor and Mayoress of Worthing, Stan and Daphne Moore, the MP for Worthing, Terence Higgins and the Chairman of West Sussex County Council, Peter Shepherd and Mrs. Shepherd together with Council representatives.

The flower arrangements in lemon and peach colours caught the Princess's eye as she entered the Day Centre where she was officially welcomed to St Barnabas' by the Chairman, Mr. Wilfred East and his wife, Carol. Dr. Kingsbury conducted the Princess around the administration area, introducing members of staff and pointing out to her the portrait of Dr. Gusterson. In the new Day Centre, she unveiled a plaque which read: 'To commemorate the visit of H.R.H. The Princess of Wales. November 29,1985'. She signed an official portrait – Diana – in her well known style and also the Home's visitors' book. She then chatted with some of the helpers and staff, and made private visits to the wards. At a buffet lunch, she was able to have further informal conversations. Many people recall with delight the impact of her visit. The Hon Chaplain, the Revd Hugh Ford, was struck by the way in which she remembered so much about the individual patients to whom she had spoken. The cook, Joy Watts, discovered that the Princess' favourite dessert was cold tapioca and jam – and then explained to her the culinary aspects of bacon roly-poly which the Princess had never come across. (Joy is now on her third kitchen, having joined St Barnabas' 25 years ago as a ward orderly but who was asked by Miss Sackse to work in the kitchen 'temporarily' as she had forgotten that she had hired her!) And one patient, just after Princess Diana had

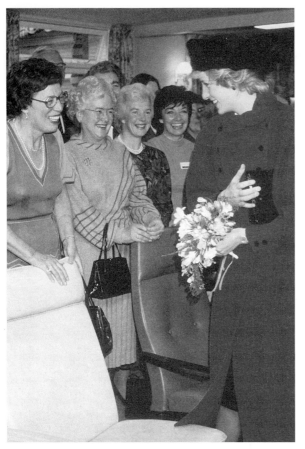

13 *Diana, Princess of Wales, meets a group of volunteers. (Photo:* Worthing Herald*)*

spoken to her said, 'If I had to die now, I should die happy'. At the end of her visit, the Princess went on one of her famous walkabouts to talk with the schoolchildren who were waiting outside in the cold rain. Altogether, a memorable visit by this sunny Princess.

Dr. Kingsbury decided to retire from the post of Medical Director in March 1993. Looking back on 16 very important years in his life, he wrote:

> Time spent with the patient and their family and friends was the essence, listening to the patient, hearing what they were saying, listening to what they were saying with their hearts and minds not just what was on their lips.

Whilst we have not looked at all the activities during his leadership, the development of the four main aspects of his vision for St Barnabas' has been described. He was Medical Director for 12 years, and had lately suffered much back pain which had demanded hospital treatment. This chapter has tried to show the immensity of his contribution to the life and work of St Barnabas'. It was a time of fast, extensive growth, of activity in unexplored areas of care and of being bold enough to take the necessary risks. Under his guidance St Barnabas' had been enlarged and expanded so that it had become a Hospice which was, and still is, much admired.

But for the second time in its history, a successor was waiting in the wings. Dr. Adrian Ruddle had joined St Barnabas' as Physician in 1987, having had experience in general practice in the UK and Australia, and hospice experience at St Gemma's Hospice, Leeds. As Physician he had been mainly concerned with the clinical responsibility of in-patients. With the closeness of his involvement with the work of St Barnabas', the Council were unanimous in offering him the post of Medical Director.

CHAPTER 5

THE CENTRE OF EXCELLENCE

We must now look at the finances of St Barnabas'. Much had happened since the first 10-shilling donation and the settlement of the cost of the original building in 1973. We have seen how the service to patients was set up and how that service developed both inside the Hospice and in the community. What were the financial implications? The situation at the end of March 1974 – the first financial year – was as follows:

Total income	£107,475
of which the main sources were	
Hospital Board	£27,198
NSCR	£6,000
Patients' fees	£27,901
Legacies	£26,299
Total expenditure	£82,238
Surplus	£25,237

This was a highly satisfactory set of results, although we have seen that fluctuations in income and expenditure during the year caused some headaches. The average cost per day to run the Home was £225. By the end of 1980, this had risen to £1,000. The Council had been worried about the nursing costs of £¼ million in the previous year but it is not so much the snapshot of the finances as the trends that are the real measure.

Dr. Gusterson had always boasted that the uniqueness of St Barnabas' was that it was entirely independent while yet receiving 'quite a large measure of financial support from the National Health Service'. He felt that this was a much healthier situation than many other Homes enjoyed which, built from private sources, nevertheless relied 100 per cent on NHS funding. In his opinion, St Barnabas' was 'able to maintain itself quite well financially'. This was not always the view of subsequent treasurers and bursars; and, although there is still funding today through the NHS, it represents approximately only 10 per cent of total expenditure.

With a requirement to be able to guarantee, as far as possible, a steady, growing income, the basic question was: to what objective should investment income be addressed? For example, at first investment income was used for current expenditure, and in 1977 the Council felt they should instead concentrate on capital growth. That decision would itself be determined by whether they should be protecting capital or considering the need for expansion. This was at a time when income from legacies and donations had nearly doubled since the previous year and the high interest rates meant that interest on deposit had risen substantially. By February 1978 the value of investments was about £250,000 and in March 1979 £320,000.

In considering sources of income, the Council tried to remain open to ideas, such as a proposition circulated by a firm of stockbrokers, Messrs Buckmaster & Moore, that a Cancer Care Unit Trust should be established, people subscribing in the ordinary way and the income given to a group of cancer charities. The Council's view was that, however attractive the scheme might be, it might alienate some existing subscribers and be counter-productive.

Investments played an important part in financing. In 1975, the market value of their Stock Exchange securities was £13,567, and included, besides Treasury Stock, ordinary shares in Estates and Agency Holdings, The Guthrie Corporation, LRC International, P & O, The Rank Organisation, Bristol Plant Ltd., English China Clays, Barratt Development Ltd., Marley Ltd, Holt Products and Tesco Stores. In May of the following year the investments were valued at £49,600. In order to increase the income from these investments, all the equity shares were sold and were re-invested in Treasury Stock. In October 1976 the investments were valued at £72,900; in May two years later this had risen to £293,566 and the Hon. Treasurer, Mr. Cuming, recommended that they should be looked after professionally, either by brokers or through a bank. The prompt decisions needed in a volatile market were causing an unacceptable workload on the finance staff. The Council appointed Grieveson Grant & Co., Brokers, to handle their portfolio, stipulating that a partner from the company should attend a specially convened meeting of the Council to discuss the handling of the Council's investments during each year.

It is at this stage that an important trend began to emerge, the part played by legacies towards the income of St Barnabas'. These figures show their importance:

	Expenditure	Income received from legacies (per cent)
1979	£227,538	36.5
1984	£418,754	58.9
1989	£1,087,771	66.5
1994	£2,274,496	54.0
1997	£2,431,942	42.8

The costs, increasing by over 1000 per cent in 18 years, have been broadly in line with other hospices. The growth is far greater than inflation due to the expansion of patient care in the Hospice and in the community (see Fig.1 Appendix I). Legacy income is by definition volatile (see Fig.3 Appendix I). Generally legacies have enabled St Barnabas' to balance its books with a surplus each year with the alarming exception of 1995 when a severe drop in legacy income led to a £321,000 deficit. Income from legacies is not always realised immediately because, for example, where a property has been left in a will, the time taken to dispose of it may be governed by the presence of a sitting tenant. But, as Dr. Kingsbury once pointed out, the benefits received from legacies were due in no small way to local solicitors who have kept the needs of St Barnabas' in mind when clients' wills are being drawn up. The bottom line is:

without the necessarily unreliable legacy stream, the Hospice would never be able to cope financially (*see* Fig.2 Appendix I). Hence there is the need for a pro-active approach, for continuous fund-raising to secure the future and to improve and increase patient services.

This is where the role of the charity shops has become so important. In March 1987 the House Committee first considered this concept, stimulated by the advent of a Cancer Research shop in Worthing town centre. They approached this organisation who gave some useful advice which the Committee considered; the chief being that they always took a long lease on their premises, only handled good quality items and were staffed by volunteers. The possible viability for St Barnabas' was discussed,

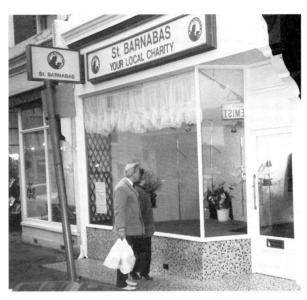

14   *The first shop, Rowlands Road, Worthing*

together with various locations, as a result of which Mr. de Beer began a feasibility study. He circulated members with two documents – 'Fund Raising' and 'Charity Shop Feasibility Study'. Committee members were very much in favour of the idea of a charity shop, the Council agreed, favouring acquiring leased premises and they instructed the House Committee to enter into negotiations.

One of the critical assumptions was that a good nucleus of volunteers would be available and be prepared to man the shop on a rota basis under the supervision of a full-time manager. In due course, completion took place on 16 November 1988 for premises in Rowlands Road, Worthing, and Mrs. Diane Byrne was recruited to run the shop, which was in fair condition but needed internal decorations in order for it to be ready to open in mid-January. The shop was officially opened by the Mayor of Worthing, Councillor John Cotton, in January, 1989 and within a very short while had established itself and was trading above the target figure set for its performance. The shop was initially financed from the Home's funds but it was expected that the loan would be repaid within the first year's trading.

Mrs. Byrne, expressing the hope that the shop would be successful and a further means of contributing to the long-term funding of St Barnabas', said:

> It was with some trepidation we opened our doors each morning for the first few weeks, fortunately we were lucky enough to get away to a good start and even more important, have been able to maintain turnover in excess of our expectations. This relative success as with so many other aspects of St Barnabas' could not have been achieved without the splendid help and enthusiasm of our Shop Volunteers. Without them the degree of funding would be considerably reduced and the spirit of the Shop completely changed.

By March, the impact of the shop on the management team was being noticed, both Dr. Kingsbury and Mr. de Beer feeling that they were being drawn away from their responsibilities for the Home. A committee was therefore set up, reporting directly to the Council, to oversee the shop; the volunteers would still be recruited

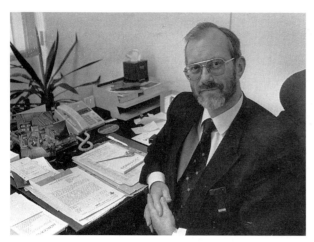

15 *Dr. Adrian Ruddle, appointed Medical Director, 1993*

by the volunteer co-ordinator and the shop manageress. (Mr. de Beer was once amused to receive a letter addressed to 'The Bertha, St Barnabus Hospital'!)

The appointment of Mrs. Penny Eggebrecht as Voluntary Services Co-ordinator in September 1988 showed how the Council were placing their trust in the volunteers to realise the potential which the shop offered. Indeed, by 1990 there were about 250 volunteers, and it was therefore possible to acquire further shop premises. The Lancing shop was opened by Derek Jameson in 1990: Rustington followed in 1991 and Storrington in 1993. These have been joined by shops in Steyning, Ferring (which specialises in used furniture), and Shoreham. In 1997, the shops raised 18 per cent of the income of St Barnabas' through the efforts of the shop managers and their 300 volunteers. With an additional 300 working at the Hospice itself, their highly significant contribution can be appreciated, both in terms of the monetary value of their time and skills and of the way in which they bring the message of St Barnabas' to the public eye.

Contributions from benefactors – individuals, associations, businesses – have continued to flow in to St Barnabas'. The sister of a former patient, herself a pensioner, made over 200 Corn Dollies which raised over £100. Dolls of another kind were the province of Miss Queenie Butler from Goring, who specialised in dressing 21in. dolls using continental materials, silk and lace which she received from her god-daughter. Queenie's dolls became legendary as raffle prizes and the Hospice has benefited by thousands of pounds through her work. Following a Gala Evening at the Connaught Theatre, the Worthing Ladies Circle presented a cheque for £300. Six children from the John Selden School held a sponsored silence, raising £94. Sometimes the gifts were in kind. The Sussex Bar Billiards Association gave an electric ironing machine; in 1981, Datsun offered to meet the cost of installing gas-fired central heating. Nissan continued their enthusiastic support by paying for new uniforms for the nursing Staff at a cost of £4,500 and a year later they met the £20,000 cost of re-flooring for the wards. The Worthing Rotary Club sponsored an appeal for £13,500 to purchase a minibus, which they handed over in October 1988; the bus gave ten years' sterling service. (One unexpected advantage of the minibus came when the shire horse 'Brigadier', with his wagon, was brought on a visit to the Hospice. The hoist on the minibus was used to raise patients in their wheelchairs so that they could better inspect 'Brigadier's' noble features.)

The previous year, the Administrator reported that the Hospice had received 'donations for specific purposes, such as a new, secure medicine trolley, word processor, £700 worth of shrubs and plants, a fountain and a franking machine'.

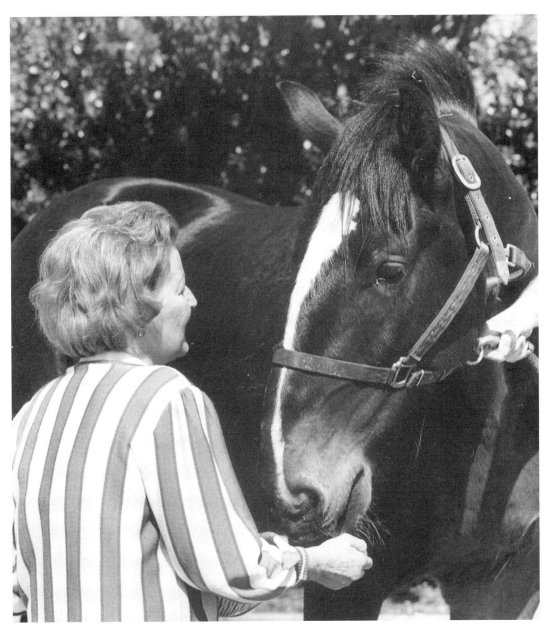

16 *Lavinia, the President, makes friends with 'Brigadier' the shire horse*

He termed some of this support 'valiant', quoting PC Stapleton of Worthing who had run a half-marathon, walked 25 miles and cycled 50 miles all in one day, raising £1,300, and a lady in Upper Beeding who had stopped smoking and raised over £1,000 from that effort.

But one of the most popular fund-raising events has always been the annual fête. The first was proposed for 29 June 1974 but owing to a short planning period it was not possible to hire a marquee (it was impracticable to hold the event in the Home).

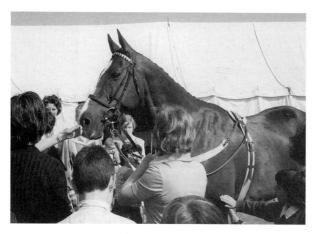

17 'Aldaniti', star guest at the fête

Instead, a Sale was held in St Paul's Church Hall on 2 October at which nearly £700 was raised (over £4,000 at 1998 values). The first fête held at St Barnabas' was on 18 June 1975. There was a profit of £1,050, which was judged to be 'an excellent result and a most welcome addition' to the finances and the Bursar was reported to 'be smiling ever since'. Many relatives and friends of past patients attended, much to everyone's delight. The patients were also involved; one lady, who had no outdoor clothes with her, sent for her fur coat and went out three times during the afternoon to look round the stalls. In 1976, in spite of unkind weather, the total raised was £1,250; the next year this rose to £1,543. In addition to being a fund-raiser the fête was becoming 'quite a social affair', as Dr. Gusterson put it; it was an opportunity to keep in touch with friends and to meet many relatives, as well as patients who had been at St Barnabas' and were now home again. On these sound foundations the fête has flourished, thanks to the incredible amount of work put in by volunteers, committee members and the staff. In 1983, when the sum raised was almost £5,000, this was the first time that there had been an admission charge (which led to a long queue forming down Columbia Drive) but around 1,000 people attended. There were two special attractions – the visit of Lady Colwyn who brought her vintage Rolls Royce (much to the interest of the men and boys) and of 'Aldaniti', the winner of the 1981 Grand National. He proved a great attraction as he paraded in front of the marquees. The fête continues to be popular and an important source of income.

Another of the public faces of St Barnabas' is the float which is entered at the Worthing Carnival. Whether the subject is 'Batman' or 'Cinderella', the float has a splendid reputation for carrying off the first prize. Success in the Adur Bath Tub Race has been more elusive. Indeed, part of the ethos of the Hospice is its great sense of fun. The photograph albums show patients and staff relaxing and enjoying themselves – whether at the 21st Anniversary Ball or the shows and parties held throughout the year – another sign of its family atmosphere.

One far-reaching decision made by the Council as a result of the fall in legacy income was to promote the formation of the Friends of St Barnabas' groups in order to publicise the work of the Hospice in towns and villages. As we have seen, individuals and small groups have given continuing fund-raising support throughout its history, but with the formation of the Friends, this could be channelled and enhanced. Within the first year, the groups raised over £30,000 and amply justified the Council's confidence. One local group, led by Lucy Tricker and her brother Richard from East Preston, consists solely of teenagers.

There has always been a strong religious emphasis in the life of St Barnabas' though not in a sectarian sense; at one stage, Dr. Gusterson had commented that he

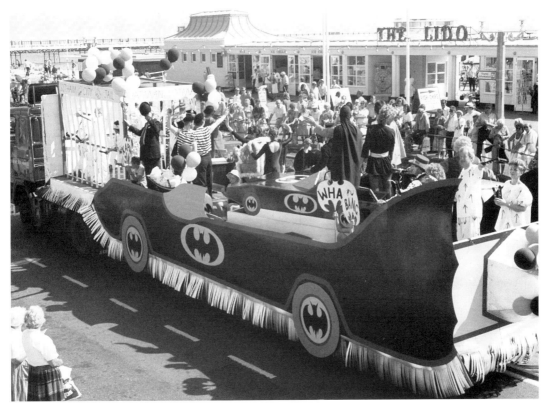

18 *The 'Batman' float, Worthing Carnival, 1994*

had counted 26 different religions or denominations amongst the patients over the years, including 'some of the more unusual faiths. Great tact had to be exercised in dealing with the subject of religion'. An altar was placed in a recess in the Day Room, with a 6ft. by 3ft. ceramic altar piece of unusual design. From the beginning there was a weekly service of Holy Communion on Tuesdays, using a booklet designed by Dr. Gusterson. Being held in the Day Room it was possible for patients to be non-participating observers, if they so wished. The first Confirmation was held on 15 October 1974. Evening prayers were offered daily for the patients and staff. There was no chaplain to the Home because, as Dr. Gusterson said in 1979, this encouraged all local clergy to visit St Barnabas'.

One priest who gave his time and talents for ten years was the Revd Hugh Ford. He had extensive experience in hospital chaplaincies and visited St Barnabas' two or three times a week in his retirement. He conducted the first wedding at St Barnabas', of a very ill patient who had lived with his partner in Shoreham for many years. Mr. Ford produced a book of 'Holy Ho-Ho's' of amusing incidents from his long ministry; the sale of these helped to support the education effort by funding a staff member to attend a course in America. Perhaps it is not surprising that a nurse should comment: 'We like Mr. Ford because he cheers us all up'. When Mr. Ford retired, Dr. Kingsbury put forward the idea of a team of local clergy to provide a chaplaincy service. They were five in number, led by Revd Brian Fitzpatrick, Minister of Offington Park Methodist Church. But in 1994, by one of those strange quirks of life, four of them were to leave during a three-month period, so Mr. Fitzpatrick strongly advocated the appointment of a full-time Chaplain and Dr. Ruddle told the Council that 'the job of Hospice Chaplain takes a special type of spiritual care and calls for somebody with the right personality and experience'; without a Chaplain, they might 'not be recognised as providing a full service' to patients. Fr John McCormack took up the post in 1995.

Bricks and mortar must now claim our attention. (*See* Appendix 2. The numbers in brackets in the text refer to the numbers shown on the plan.) One of the most remarkable aspects of St Barnabas' is that as its services grew, thus creating demands for more space and facilities, at no time did the Council ever have to take out any loan to fund building works. The saving in interest payments alone is significant.

The first extension (1) was needed as early as 1974, to provide an office for Dr. Kay, the Bursar and a storeroom, being completed in August for around £8,000. At the same time double doors were installed in both wards so that beds and wheelchairs could be taken out onto the patio. The next major item was the provision of screening around the site so that the building and the mortuary could be shielded from the adjoining houses. The House Committee Minutes about this item are a classic example of Parkinson's Law. Whilst the external appearance was extremely important, they did not want to spend money which would be far better used for patient care. After a seven-month correspondence with the Worthing Borough Council, it was finally agreed to install a 6ft. concrete post and wooden panel fence at a cost of around £5,300. (This was immediately nicknamed 'Stalag XIII' by some of the staff! To add insult to injury, in the following September a lorry ploughed into the fence by the front entrance. The repairs were effected and the account settled but the two insurance companies were left 'arguing between themselves about this claim'.) When the foundations for a new store were being excavated in May 1976 the digger cut the 1in. main gas intake pipe to the Home, and the Gas Board had to be called to repair it.

At the same time extra staff changing and locker facilities were provided and it was decided to install double glazing in the wards at a cost of £3,300. This made a marked improvement to the temperature in the Home. A conversion to gas central heating was carried out for reasons of better economy and greater flexibility; the cost was £34,500. A committee room was built in 1982 (3) with additional toilets and an extension to the laundry. In 1985, (4) the Day Room was extended, and other facilities on A Wing. The condition of the flat roof had been giving some concern since the summer of 1985. The Council did consider replacing it with a pitched roof but the extra weight which this would have created might not have been supportable by the foundations (owing to the very wet nature of the original site); it would have greatly reduced the amount of light to the central area of the Home. The extensive repair work was carried out with a guarantee period up to the year 2010.

1991/2 saw a three-phase building programme which further extended the Day Room and provided a canopy for the front entrance, greatly facilitating patient and ambulance access. (A comment was heard from within a group of nurses in the Staff Room studying the builders' bare torsos: 'No, I don't think I'm that desperate'!) The second phase saw the provision of lecture and seminar rooms, accommodation for the

Home Support Unit, offices and a physiotherapy area. Phase three (5) involved alterations to existing premises but, most importantly, the conversion on Ward B to provide family rooms, so that families may be together 24 hours a day for mutual support and in privacy. Offices and storage space were the order of the day in (6) 1994, and three more family rooms and an out-patient room (7) were completed in 1997, together with a chapel. And at the heart of all this, 'Piccadilly' still remains – the place where corridors still cross, where the shop is on show and where the buzz of calm activity still prevails. And to think that the original building had no double glazing and was heated by night storage heaters!

The growth in patient care and services, and the need to provide sound financial backing has inevitably led to an expansion of support services, including computer data bases, information technology, business planning, personnel services and fund-raising. One sign of this increased competence was the appointment of the first General Manager, Alan Welton, in 1993, as were later appointments of a Fund-raising Co-ordinator and a Retail Co-ordinator to help the shops. There are some who may feel that there is too much emphasis on 'running a business', but to use that word pejoratively would be to err because, although the total nursing, medical and administrative staff now numbers 131, care and comfort and consolation are still at the very heart of St Barnabas'. It is appropriate that we should focus on that for our final comments.

The experienced nursing team, still with a ratio of 1.7 nurses to each bed, exhibits the same skills that have always given St Barnabas' its reputation as a centre of excellence. They still show the ability to listen, to have strength of character in times of considerable stress and all the time are following training programmes, whether the Diploma in Palliative Care (validated by Brighton University) or NVQ courses and study days, to increase skills and specialities. Exchanges of nurses with local hospitals are also part of the training. The eight-strong Community Palliative Care Team enjoys working relationships with GPs and district nurses which would have been the envy – and delight – of Dr. Gusterson. The Social Work department is completely involved in all aspects of Hospice care and especially in the important area of bereavement.

The Day Hospice, in welcoming patients for a day or part of a day, assists both them and their carers with programmes which include physiotherapy, reflexology, aromatherapy and the restful atmosphere of the snoezelen; recently, a lymphodema treatment service has been added. (Nor must we forget Cosworth, the black and white cat who 'dropped in' – and stayed. He gives his own brand of comfort to patients and visitors by day and night. He developed a tumour on a rear leg which had to be amputated, so he has experienced St Barnabas' care at first paw!)

Thanks to the support from Artability, a non-profit making organisation which gives people with disabilities the opportunity to participate in the arts, the striking mural to celebrate the 21st anniversary was

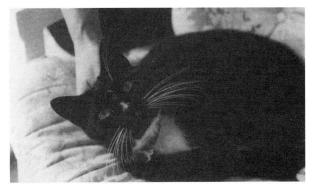

19 *Cosworth*

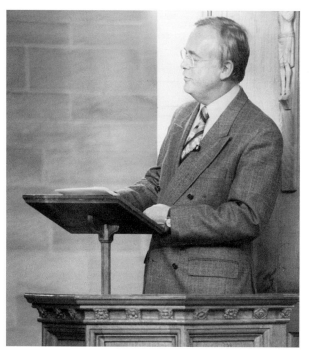

20 *Martyn Lewis gives the address at the 25th anniversary service at Lancing College*

created and graces the wall by the entrance; in 1996, the 60-page book *Blowing a Lapwing's Egg*, another of their successes, was launched at the Brighton Festival with authors and their relatives present. On the medical side, the Royal Colleges have recognised the post-graduate training posts which St Barnabas' provides and which some regard as the jewel in the crown on the educational side.

Past successes – in its 25 years, St Barnabas' has cared for over 11,000 patients. The future suggests that its capacity to care and comfort will increasingly be needed. This will demand a pro-active approach in dealing with physical, mental or spiritual distress; in providing family support, especially with children. This is likely to receive governmental encouragement especially in involvement much earlier in the treatment process. That has implications on resources and finance, and also on the present building and site.

However, no hospice today need be an island. There are increasing links with other hospices and much closer liaison with the Health Authority and local hospitals to plan for the future. The Calman Hine Report and the National Council for Hospice and Specialist Palliative Care Services (of which Dr. Ruddle is an elected member) have had a significant impact on the delivery of patient care. A more professional approach is evident as some very significant strategic decisions are faced.

In January 1998 a service of thanksgiving and celebration was held in the Chapel of Lancing College. As the story of the Hospice was read and candles were lit for each of its 25 years, the impact of its successes became clear. The broadcaster, Martyn Lewis, in his address spoke of this story and gave his own creed for the Hospice movement, of which the first statement was: 'We will give you nothing less than the finest quality of care to be found in the British Isles'. St Barnabas', with its 'life-raft of Hospice services' still had the 'opportunity to help countless more families throughout West Sussex'.

One suspects that its founder, the 'doctor, partridge plump', whose vision it was, would, if present, have smiled in approval with a twinkle in his eye.

APPENDIX I

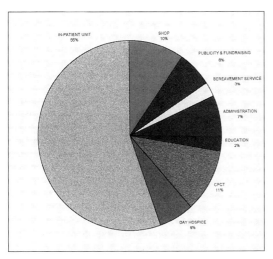

Fig.1 *Expenditure 1996/7*   **Fig.2** *Sources of Income 1996/7*

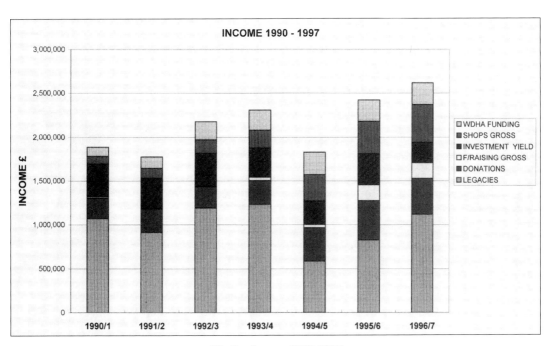

Fig.3 *Income 1990-1997*

APPENDIX II

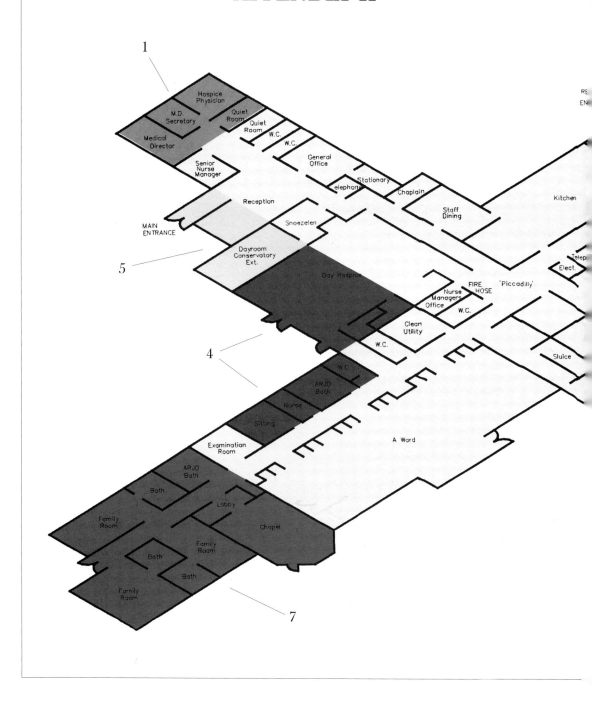

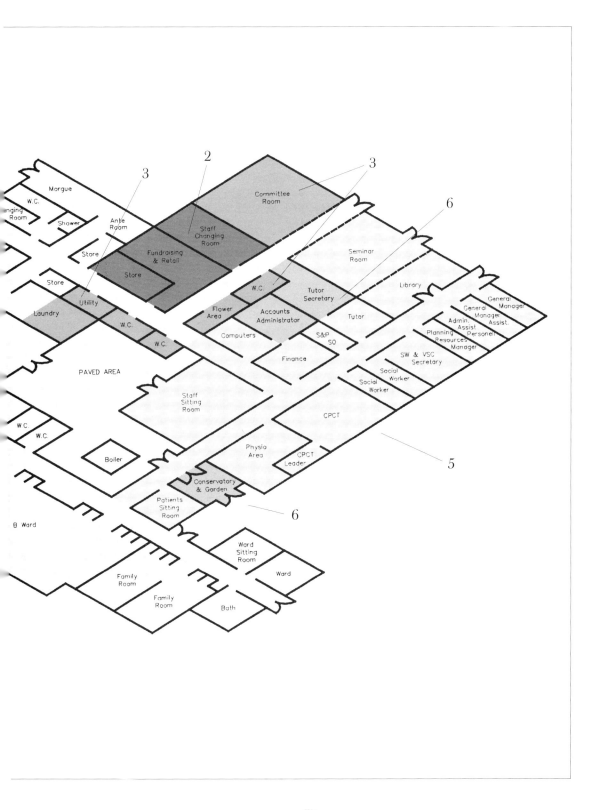

APPENDIX III

Presidents

1968-1975 ..... Bernard, 16th Duke of Norfolk
1975-1995 ..... Lavinia, Duchess of Norfolk
1995- .... Lady Sarah Clutton

Chairmen of Council

1973-1984 ..... Mr. B.W.F. Roe
1984-1988 ..... Mr. E.W. East
1988-1992 ..... Mrs. P. Bowles
1992-1995 ..... Dr. P.C. Reynolds
1995- .... Mrs. J. Annis

Medical Directors

1973-1981 ..... Dr. F.R. Gusterson
1981-1993 ..... Dr. A.W. Kingsbury
1993- .... Dr. A. Ruddle

Matrons

1973-1975 ..... Miss F. Sackse
1975-1988 ..... Miss M.E. Stroud
1988-1989 ..... Miss M. Chapman
1989-1996 ..... Miss H. Fittock
1996- .... Mrs S. Mason (Senior Nurse Manager)

INDEX

Alvey, Mrs. D., 4
Amberley Young Wives, 19
Artability, 53-4

Barrass, J.C., 42
Bedford, J., 3
Beecham's Research Laboratories, 4, 13
Berry, E., 29
Bird, E. Manley, 3
Blowing a Lapwing's Egg, 54
Board, Lillian, 8
Bollom, Mrs., 17
Bower, Sandra, 13
Bowles, Mrs. P., 41-3
Bradwell, H.C., 17, 23, 29
Buckmaster & Moore, 46
Bunce, H.T., 3, 9, 11, 12, 16, 21
Burton, S., 19
Butler, Miss Q., 48
Byrne, Mrs. D., 47

Caddick, T., 38-9
Caer Gwent Nursing Home, 1
Calman Hine Report, 54
Chapman, Miss M., 37
Cheal & Sons, 10
Clutton, Lady Sarah, 28
Colwyn, Lady, 50
Cosworth, 53
Cotton, Cllr. J., 47
Cox, Mrs. A., 42
CRUSE, 39
Cuming, C.E., 46
Cummings, Miss R., 35

Datsun, 48
Davey, E.C., 17
de Beer, F., 42, 47-8
Deutsch, Dr. G., 30
Diana, H.R.H. Princess of Wales, 43
Durrington Townswomen's Guild, 13

East, E.W., 40, 43
East Sussex Area Health Authority, 27
Eggebrecht, Mrs. P., 48

Evans, N., 6
Evans, Revd. N., 25

Fittock, Miss H., 37, 39
Fitzpatrick, Revd. B., 52
Flower Fund, 1
Ford, Revd. H., 43, 51
Frampton, H., 15
Francis, Dr. R.E., 1, 3, 29
Franklin, Mrs. J., 42
Franks, Dr. R.B., 1, 3, 29

Gilbey, J.A., 3
Gisby, E., 6, 31
Goatcher & Son, 19
Gray, Sister M., 39
Grieveson Grant & Co, 46
Grose, Sister C., 39
Guild Care, 1
Gusterson, Mrs. D., 12, 32
Gusterson, Dr. F.R.: invitation to chair appeal, 1-2; career, 2; appeal launch, 4; opposition, 6; site, 7-8; building, dedication service, 8-12; medical director, 10, 17-33; fund-raising, 13-16; official opening, 19; links with local GPs, 26-7; links with other units, 30-1; overseas visitors, 31; education, 31; Christian faith, 31, 33-4, 50-1; awarded Cross of Honour, 33; retirement and death, 33-4; 40, 45, 50, 53

Hammond, K., 42
Harvey-Samuel, Cdr. and Mrs. J., 34
Hazelden, Staff Nurse J., 35
Heene Road Medical Practice, 26
Heptinstall, Sister D., 25, 35
Higgins, Hon. T., 43
Hunnibal, C., 4
Hunter, Mrs. J., 42-43

Iggleden, Monsignor A.C., 5
Independent Order of Foresters, 15

Jameson, D., 48
Janisch, Revd. H., 3, 5, 10
John Selden School, 48

Kay, Dr. J., 22, 25-6, 52
Keeling, H., 2-3, 9
Kingsbury, Dr. A.: 30, 33; medical director, 33-44; education, 37-9; home care, 39-40; volunteers, 40-2; day centre, 42-4; legacies, 46; shops, 47

Lancing College, 54
Lawson, Sister E., 39
Lephard, Mrs. N., 3-4, 40
Lewis, M., 54
Lock, P., 12
Lunt, Rt. Revd. E., 12, 23

McCormack, Revd. J., 52
McNeil, D., 13, 15
Macrae, Mrs. L., 42
Maskell, Mrs. M., 14
Mason, The Ven. L., 5
Moore, Mr. & Mrs. S., 43
Morley, Sister H., 39

Nash, Miss, 33
National Council for Hospice and Specialist Palliative Care Services, 54
National Society for Cancer Research (N.S.C.R.), 6, 8, 9, 18, 22, 29, 30, 38, 45
Nelson, Miss I., 10
Nissan, 48
Noel Buxton Trust, 15
Norfolk, Bernard 16th Duke of, 5
Norfolk, Lavinia Duchess of, 5, 27, 34, 43

Pannett, Juliet, 33
Pennells, B., 3, 8
Peryer, Mrs. H.M., 3
Pilbeam, Miss, 10
Priory, The, 2, 5

Ramsey, Sue, 42
Reeves, Revd. Canon J.W., 3, 4, 10, 34
Regional Hospital Board, 11, 20, 21, 23, 29
Roe, B.W.F., 3, 10, 12, 15, 17, 30, 33
Roxburghe, Duchess of, 19, 21
Royal Air Force, Central Band of Women's, 14
Royal Marines, Band of, 14
Ruddle, Dr. A., 40, 44, 52, 54

St Christopher's Hospice, 5, 19, 25, 31
St John's Ambulance Brigade, 12
St John's Church, Worthing, 13
St Mary's Church, Storrington, 34
St Mary's Church, Thakeham, 15, 16, 21
St Paul's Church, Worthing, 12, 34, 50
Sackse, Miss F., 10, 22, 25, 43
Saunders, Dr. (later Dame) Cicely, 5, 25
Sayers, J., 1, 2, 7
Shepherd, Mr. & Mrs. P., 43
Sloss, W., 15
Snelling, J.C., 43
Southlands Hospital, 10
Stapleton, PC, 49
Stapleton, R.V., 3, 16
Stroud, Miss M., 25, 34-6
Sun Alliance, 17, 19
Sussex Bar Billiards Association, 48
Swandean Hospital, 6

Taylor, Mrs. J., 43
Temperance Building Society, 10, 19
Tricker, Lucy & Richard, 50

Ward, Maj-Gen. Sir Philip, 43
Watts, J., 19
Watts, Mrs. J., 43
Welton, A., 53
West Chiltington Flower Club, 15
West Nova Scotia Regt., 15
West Sussex County Council, 5, 8
West Sussex Nursing Homes Association, 6
West Sussex Players, 14
West Sussex Travel Society, 11
Withers, Mr., 19
Worthing Borough Council, 52
Worthing Boys' Club, 2
Worthing Companions Club, 15
Worthing Council for Social Service, 1, 2
Worthing & District Ladies Auxiliary League, 5
Worthing Gazette, 5, 8, 13
Worthing Herald, 6, 7, 13
Worthing Hospital Management Committee, 3
Worthing Inner Wheel, 15
Worthing Ladies Circle, 13, 48
Worthing Lions 200 Club, 15
Worthing Mayflower Club, 13
Worthing Musical Comedy Society, 15
Worthing Remembrance Fund, 1
Worthing Rotary Club, 48
Worthing Soroptimists, 15
Worthing and Southlands School of Nursing, 38
Worthing Town Council, 7, 8